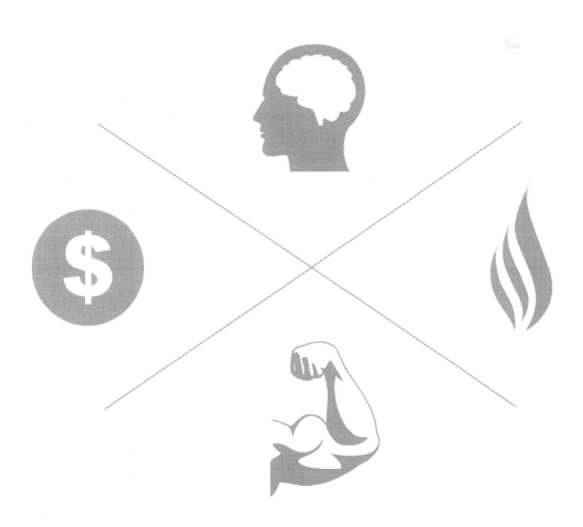

For more information about the 4 Futures Philosophy,

as well as a special video from the Authors, visit:

the4Futures.com

Introduction

You have a future in each area of your life. You're trending in a direction.
Is that direction going up?

If you're reading and using this journal for the first time, Welcome! We are honored that you've found out about us and what we are trying to do. Some people wonder, *why did you create a journal?* Over our time as business owners and coaches, we have seen many people chase dreams, only to sacrifice one part of their life to attain some type of success in another. With this in mind, we created the 4 Futures.

The 4 Futures is a philosophy where happiness, fulfillment, and success come from having success in each of these 4 areas: Mind, Meaning, Muscle, and Money. What does that mean?

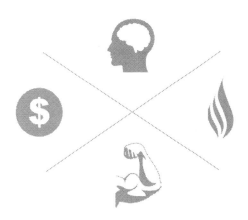

Mind

This is having a positive philosophy about the world and being able to deal with the stress of the world in a healthy way. The world is STRESSFUL - we've been around long enough to know that. When things come up, we need to deal with them in a healthy way. Sometimes that includes gaining perspective about how small our troubles are compared to a mom raising her kids in a mud hut in Haiti, or a child scrounging for food in Ethiopia. The best way we have found to deal with this is to practice mindfulness and gratitude everyday. We have also found that daily journaling of three things you appreciate greatly helps with maintaining a positive perspective. As for mindfulness, we suggest doing short guided, or un-guided, meditation each day. Phone apps for meditation can be helpful if you're just starting - we like Calm, 10% Happier, or Waking Up.

Meaning

Meaning is a little more of an ethereal idea. It's the idea that for us to be happy, we need to have close connections with other people and to a higher power. Studies show that connections with other people give happiness and contribute to longevity, and even Bronnie Ware wrote that one of the 5 regrets of the dying is "I wish I had stayed in touch with my friends." Also, we believe that having a relationship with a higher power is very important to living a purposeful life. Between these two areas, when we work towards 'Meaning' everyday, let's focus on developing closer relationships with those we love and with a power bigger than ourselves.

Muscle

The positive effects of keeping a healthy body are innumerable. We've all seen the effects of ageing in ourselves and others. We've also seen that when we start to focus on our own health, it doesn't impact just our muscles, it improves our outlook on life. Best efforts to work out every day, even if we are traveling or on vacation, will allow us to remain mobile and flexible while living a vibrant and healthy life. Sometimes that's 8 minutes of high intensity squats or pushups, and sometimes it's a longer run or bike ride. No matter what, we try to make it a point to sweat every day. Your health is also reliant on the food you eat, so make sure you're choosing healthy options to give you the proper fuel for energy and health.

Money

Every day we both coach business owners on efficiency and good decisions. Whether you're the owner of a business, or just the owner of YOU - you can always be working on making sure the financial picture is brighter for you in the future. Maybe that's balancing your checkbook, going to work, or maybe it's reviewing your 401k plan to make sure it's invested in the right place with the lowest fees. No matter what, every day you should do some item that helps your financial position improve in some way or another.

The beginning is the most important part of the work. - Plato

Date 1 / 6 / 20	**Today I Appreciate:**

Today I Appreciate:
1. My family, our home and our abundance
2. Our family's health, vibrancy and healthy habits
3. Personal, financial and business growth and friendships that have been created this year

Daily Priorities:

1 Journaling
Meditation (Guided)

2 J.V. Push workout/ w cardio

3 Meet w/ K.L reguarding Live Event
Morning Huddle

4 then Pt's

5 Perfomance Review S.M

6 Call w/ Billing Dept.

7 Pick-up Brady Soccer

8

9 Screens off
QT w/ L.C.

I'm strengthened knowing:
That I am a good providor for my family and they will be well taken care of regardless of what happens to me

I'm looking forward to:
Stretching the limits of possibility in personal and professional growth - and finding my own true potential.

I will enrich my future by...

- Journal
- Calm App
- 10 mins

Mind ✓

Love Bombs:
TM ✓
SK ✓
KD ✓
AM ✓

✓ Meaning

PUSH DAY:
- Chest
- Shoulders
- 5k

Muscle ✓

- Complete Loan App
- Opened Profit Accounts

✓ Money

A common theme that I'm seeing in my thought patterns...

Relationships:
-Consider creating scheduled time for out of town trips w/o boys for the quarter.
-No Screen rule after 7:00pm
-Complete Love Bombs before leaving house - 4 per day
-One-on-One activity 2x a month with boys
Reinstitute 2x/mo date night

Weekly Wrap-Up

3 great things that happened this week:

1) All practices met weekly production goals

2) Bryce got his driver's license

3) L.A. trip for Crossroads kitchen Res.

4 Futures Score Card

	M	T	W	R	F	S	S	Total 26/28
Mind	1	1	1	1	1	1	1	7 /7
Meaning	1	1	1	1	1	1	1	7 /7
Muscle	1	1	1	1	1	1	0	6 /7
Money	1	1	1	1	1	0	1	6 /7

Next week, I will improve _____ by...	One area I excelled at this week
Having ongoing list of money tasks to do outside of office.	I was able to journal and meditate 7 straight days and did a minimum of 4 love bombs / day x 7

Looking Ahead to Next Week...

Major tasks I need to work on

- Complete outline for I.S.P Book
- PPT for Summit

- 7 episodes in can
- Complete Associate Onboarding for M.S.

My theme this week is...
Efficiency!

Big events coming up that I need to prepare for:

- D.S.S
- CDS event
- L.A Trip
- L.C. Bday

I will improve my 4 Futures Score by doing the following:

- Meal Planning
- Out of office $ Tasks

In the journal I do not just express myself more openly than I could to any person; I create myself.

- Susan Sontag

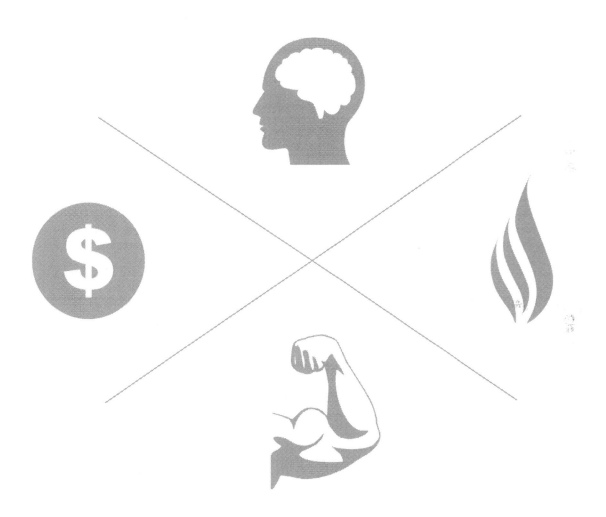

Trending and Goals

Our lives are always trending either up or down. We control what goes up or down in each by the actions we take each day. For a certain time in each of our lives, we focused too much on money, to the demise of every other area. Whether it was high times at a Wall Street bank or running small businesses, we both had times when 3 lines were trending down while the 'money' line was trending up.

Once we reset our priorities, and focused on improving our scores in each of the 4 Futures, we both found happiness and satisfaction levels that were previously unimaginable. It took practice, but it all started with a daily journal like this.

Goals

The first thing we need to do is set some long-term goals. On the next page, focus on what your life will look like in 3 years. How will your relationship be with your family? How will you react to stress? What will your health look like? And what will your financial future look like?

From there, we need to break that down into the yearly goal. In the next 12 months, what will your goals be for each area? This can be to try to improve your mindfulness practice in order to better deal with anger, it can be to try to run a mile as fast as you did in high school, or it can be to try to work with a coach to get your financial plan in order for your personal retirement or business. This can be anything, although try to make it a little bit of a stretch. Don't let yourself off too easy- while at the same time set achievable bench-marks so that you can gain good momentum.

The next step is to move down to the quarterly goals and see what you'll have to do in the next 90 days to make this yearly goal happen. If your goal is to run a mile in the same time you did in high school, then this quarter you need to just start running every other day to build up some base cardio strength. Any movement towards your goal will be great to list here.

For the last few years, we have both worked on using this exact formula every day to improve our lives, and we've seen it work in hundreds of coaching clients as well. We always coach on systems to make sure a complex organization runs well. Suffice to say that YOU are the most complex system you will ever need to manage. Managing it well is not easy, so you need to focus on the most important aspects to keeping yourself moving forward. This has worked wonders for us, and we hope it will change your life as well!

Cheers,

Alastair Macdonald

To your success,

Mark Costes, DDS

3 Year Goals...

I will experience progress and joy when...

_____

_____

_____

_____

Yearly "Big Goals" in each of the 4 Futures Category...

Mind:

Meaning:

Muscle:

Money:

To achieve my yearly goals, in 90 days I will have completed...

Mind:

Meaning:

Muscle:

Money:

The beginning is the most important part of the work. - Plato

Date ___/___/___

Daily Priorities:

1
2
3
4
5
6
7
8
9

Today I Appreciate:

1. _____
2. _____
3. _____

I'm strengthened knowing:

I'm looking forward to:

I will enrich my future by...

Mind ☐   ☐ Meaning

Muscle ☐   ☐ Money

A common theme that I'm seeing in my thought patterns...

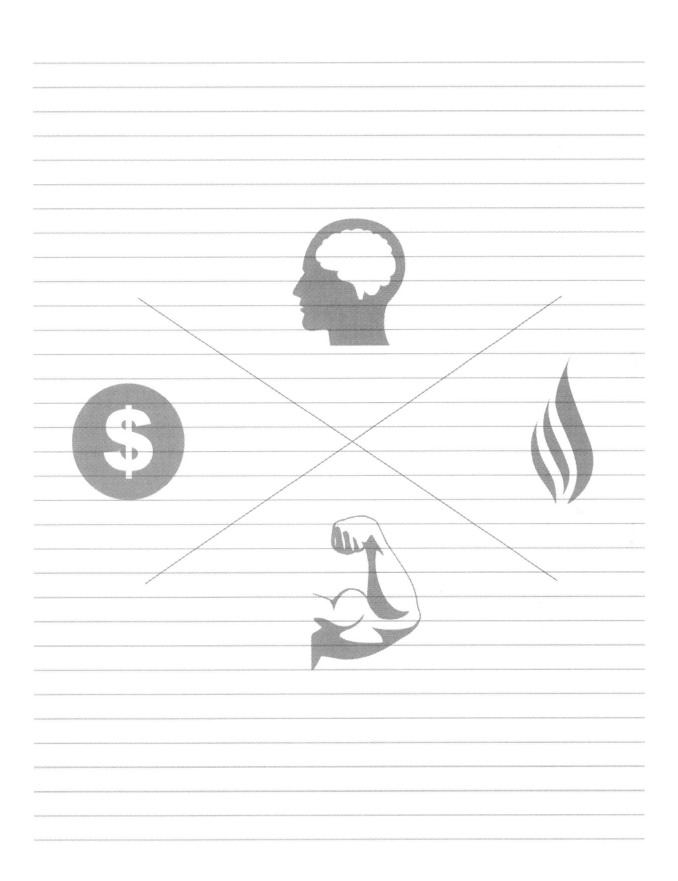

The problem with most of us, is that we would rather be ruined by praise than saved by criticism. - Norman Vincent Peale

Date _____ / _____ / _____

Daily Priorities:

1

2

3

4

5

6

7

8

9

Today I Appreciate:

1. _____

2. _____

3. _____

I'm strengthened knowing:

I'm looking forward to:

I will enrich my future by...

Mind ☐

☐ Meaning

Muscle ☐

☐ Money

A common theme that I'm seeing in my thought patterns...

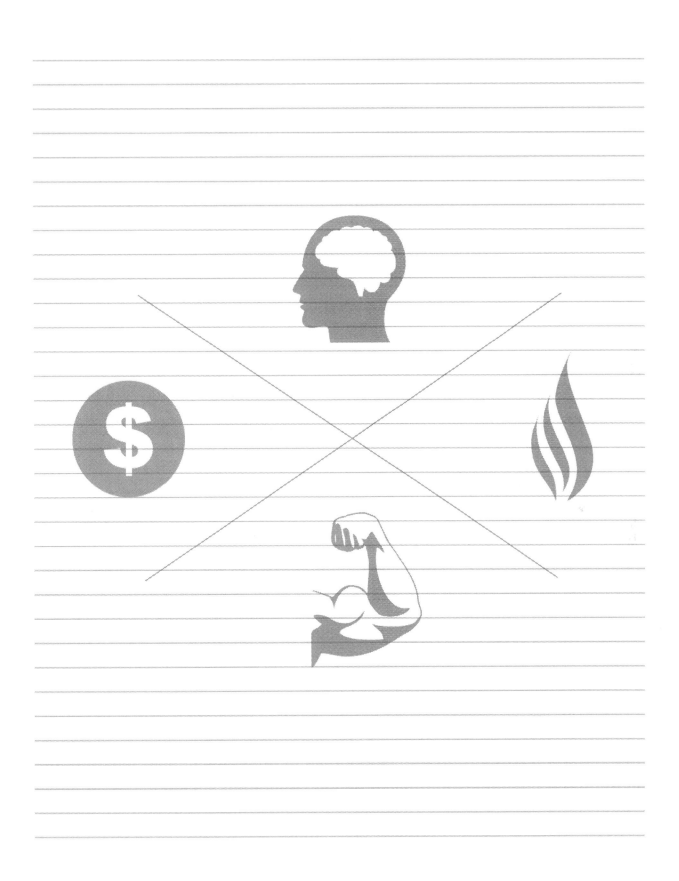

In prosperity prepare for change; in adversity hope for it. - James Burgh

Date _____ / _____ / _____

Daily Priorities:

1
2
3
4
5
6
7
8
9

Today I Appreciate:

1. _____
2. _____
3. _____

I'm strengthened knowing:

I'm looking forward to:

I will enrich my future by...

Mind ☐   ☐ Meaning

Muscle ☐   ☐ Money

A common theme that I'm seeing in relationships...

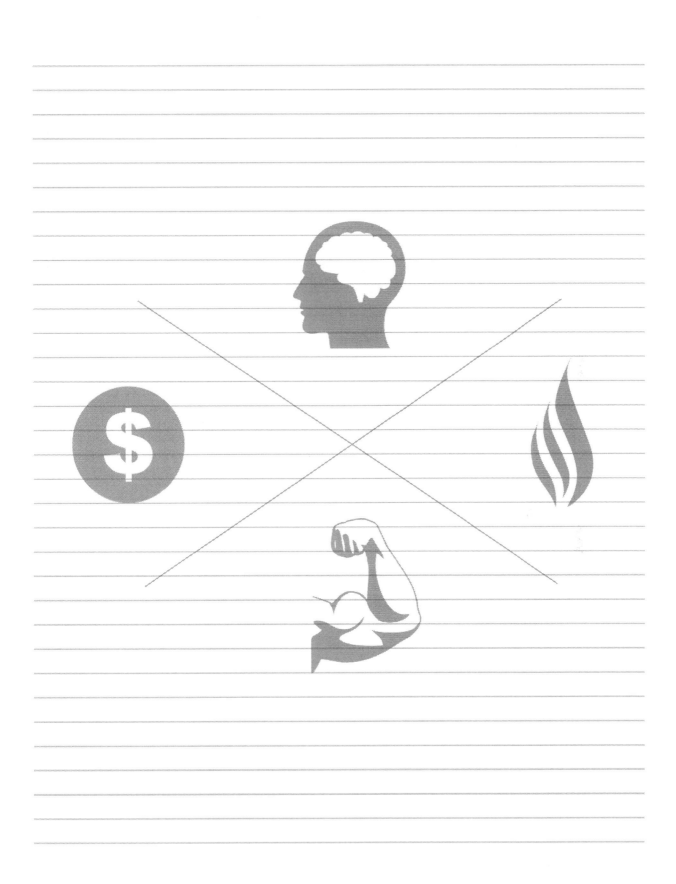

In time of change, learners inherit the earth, while the learned find themselves beautifully equipped to deal with a world that no longer exists. - Eric Hoffer

Date ___ / ___ / ___

Daily Priorities:

1
2
3
4
5
6
7
8
9

Today I Appreciate:

1. _____
2. _____
3. _____

I'm strengthened knowing:	I'm looking forward to:

I will enrich my future by...

Mind ☐   ☐ Meaning

Muscle ☐   ☐ Money

A common theme that I'm seeing in my health...

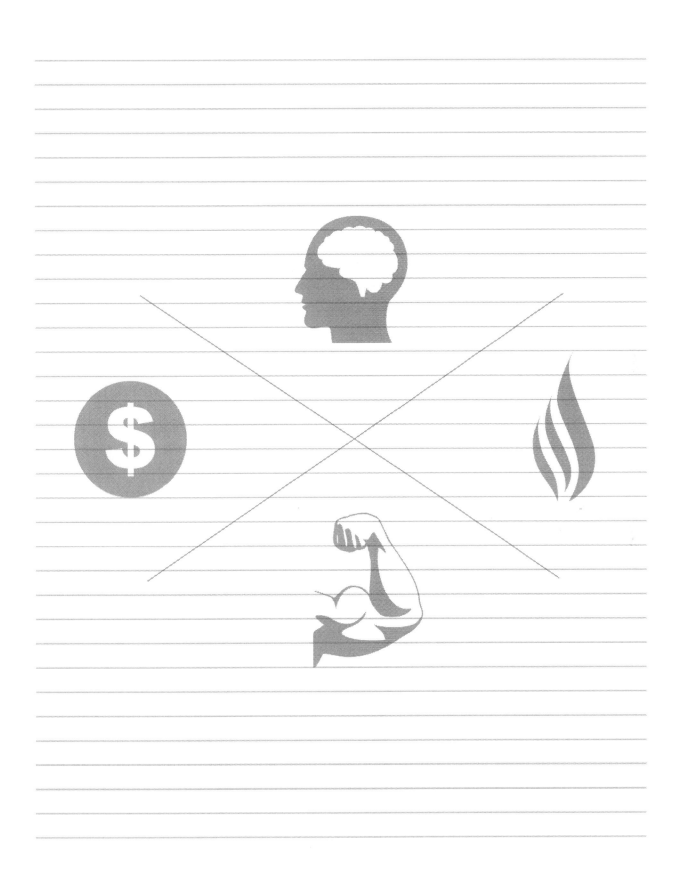

Your business, like money and power, does not build character. They reveal it. - Alastair Macdonald

Date   /   /

Daily Priorities:

1
2
3
4
5
6
7
8
9

Today I Appreciate:

1.
2.
3.

I'm strengthened knowing:

I'm looking forward to:

I will enrich my future by...

Mind ☐   ☐ Meaning

Muscle ☐   ☐ Money

A common financial theme that I'm seeing...

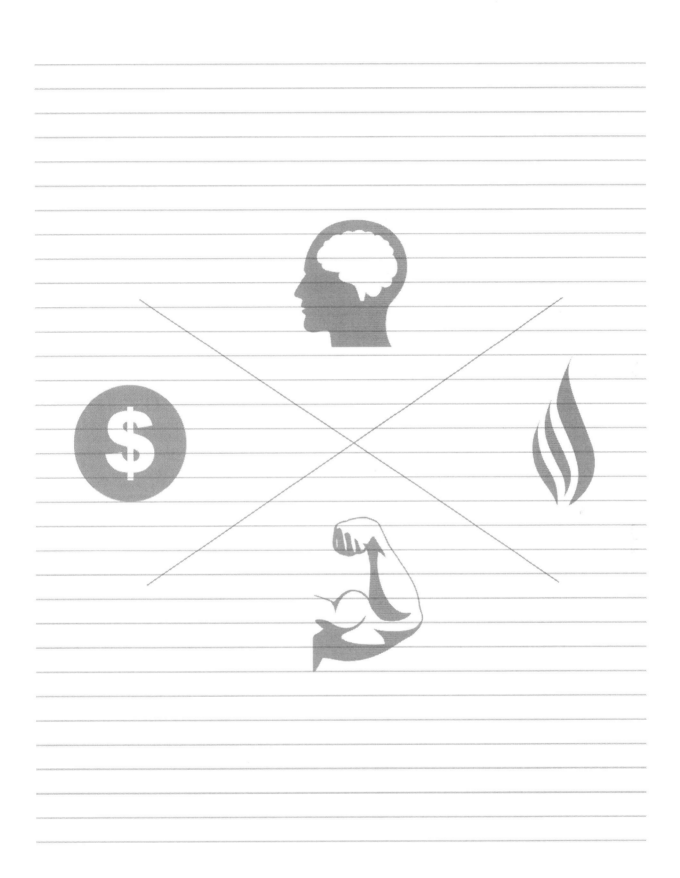

Date ___/___/___

Today I Appreciate:

1. _____

2. _____

3. _____

Daily Priorities:

1

2

3

4

5

6

7

8

9

I'm strengthened knowing:

I'm looking forward to:

I will enrich my future by...

Mind ☐

☐ Meaning

Muscle ☐

☐ Money

Something for me to contemplate with my self control...

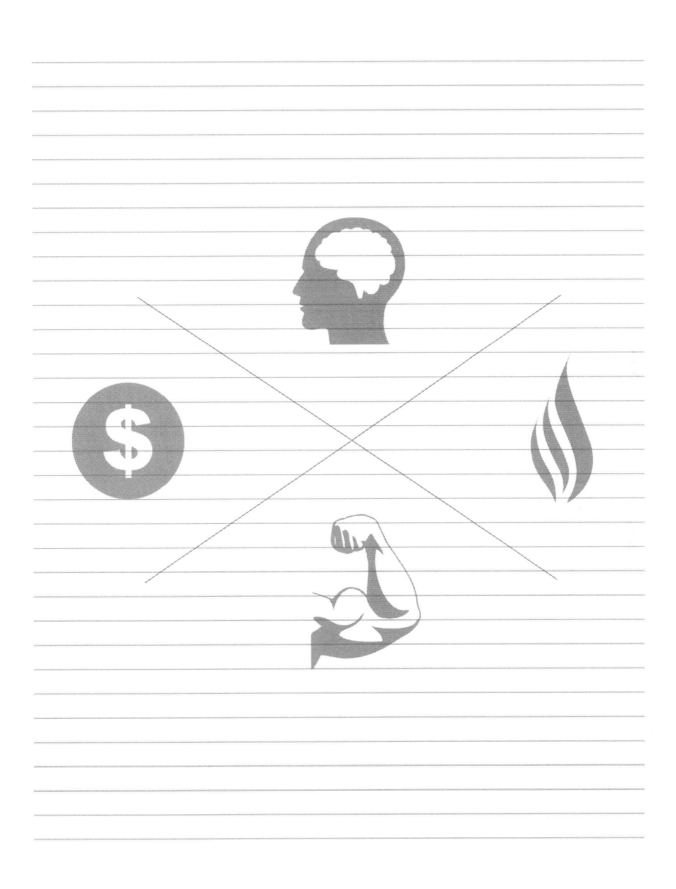

Date _____ / _____ / _____

Today I Appreciate:

1. _____

2. _____

3. _____

Daily Priorities:

1

2

3

4

5

6

7

8

9

I'm strengthened knowing:

I'm looking forward to:

I will enrich my future by...

Mind ☐

☐ Meaning

Muscle ☐

☐ Money

Something for me to contemplate in my relationships...

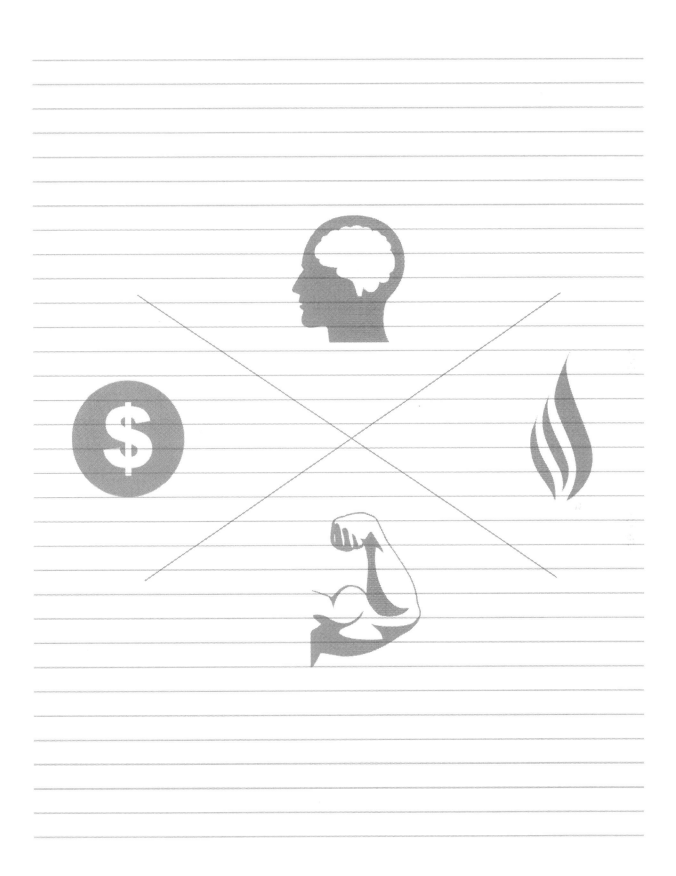

Weekly Wrap-Up

3 great things that happened this week:

_____

_____

_____

4 Futures Score Card

	M	T	W	R	F	S	S	Total	/28
Mind									/7
Meaning									/7
Muscle									/7
Money									/7

Next week, I will improve _____ by...	One area I excelled at this week

Looking Ahead to Next Week...

Major tasks I need to work on

My theme this week is...

Big events coming up that I need to prepare for:	I will improve my 4 Futures Score by doing the following:

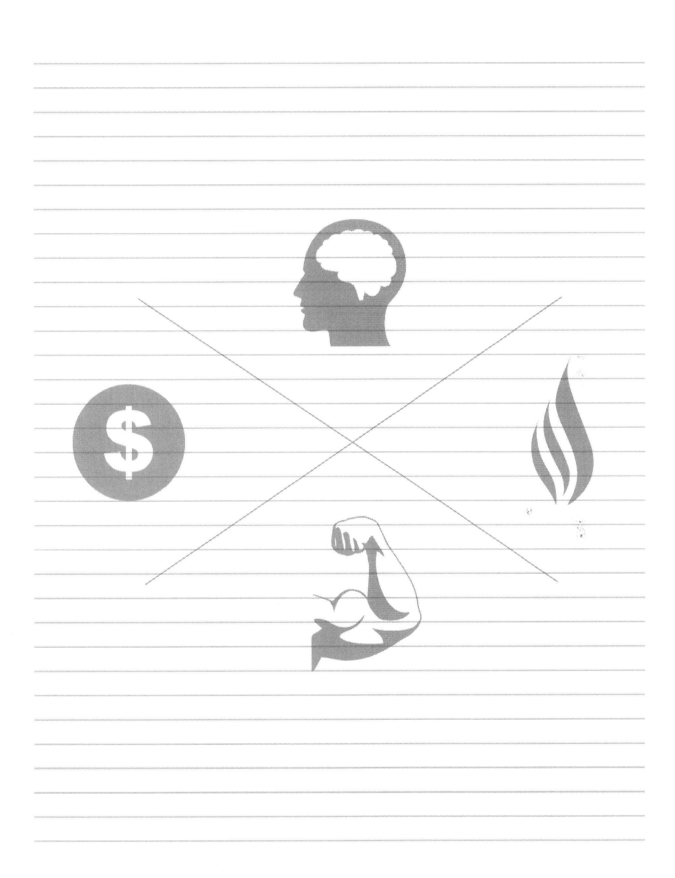

A good horse should be seldom spurred. - Thomas Fuller

Date _____ / _____ / _____

Daily Priorities:

1 ....
....
....

2 ....
....

3 ....
....

4 ....
....

5 ....
....

6 ....
....

7 ....
....

8 ....
....

9 ....
....

Today I Appreciate:

1. _____

2. _____

3. _____

I'm strengthened knowing:

I'm looking forward to:

I will enrich my future by...

Mind ☐

☐ Meaning

Muscle ☐

☐ Money

Something for me to contemplate in order to improve how I physically feel...

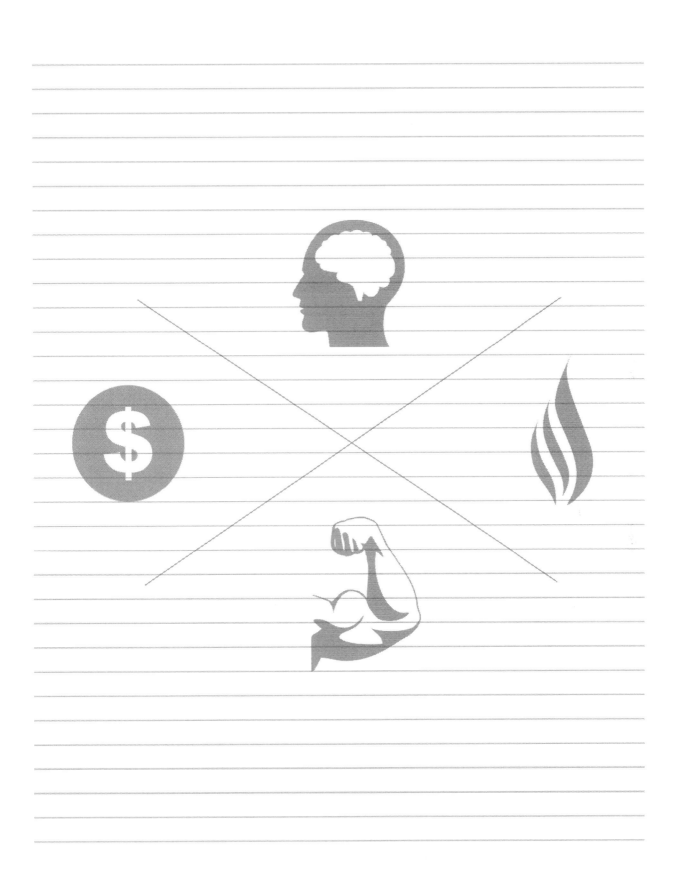

Money; (noun) A blessing that is of no advantage to us, excepting when we part with it. - Ambrose Bierce

Date _____ / _____ / _____

Today I Appreciate:

1. ....

2. ....

3. ....

Daily Priorities:

1

2

3

4

5

6

7

8

9

I'm strengthened knowing:

I'm looking forward to:

I will enrich my future by...

Mind ☐   ☐ Meaning

Muscle ☐   ☐ Money

Something for me to contemplate in order to improve my long-term financial safety would be...

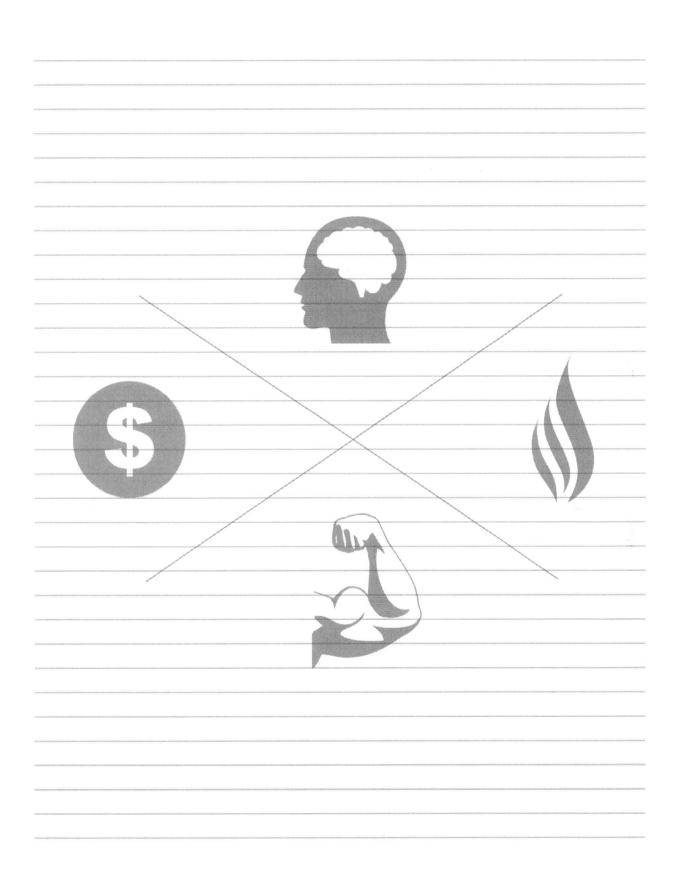

*It seems that in the advanced stages of stupidity, a lack of ideas is
compensated for by an excess of ideologies. - Carlos Ruiz Zafron*

Date ___ / ___ / ___

Daily Priorities:

1
2
3
4
5
6
7
8
9

Today I Appreciate:

1. _____
2. _____
3. _____

I'm strengthened knowing:

I'm looking forward to:

I will enrich my future by...

Mind ☐   ☐ Meaning

Muscle ☐   ☐ Money

With my mental focus, what if…

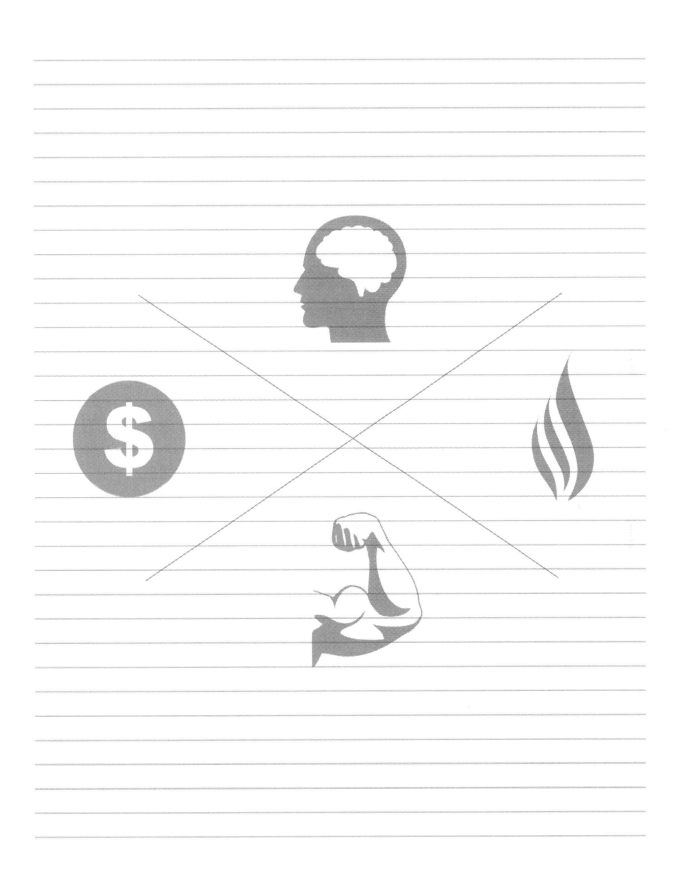

Date ___ / ___ / ___

Daily Priorities:

1 ....
2 ....
3 ....
4 ....
5 ....
6 ....
7 ....
8 ....
9 ....

Today I Appreciate:

1. _____

2. _____

3. _____

I'm strengthened knowing:

I'm looking forward to:

I will enrich my future by...

Mind ☐

☐ Meaning

Muscle ☐

☐ Money

In order to become closer to those around me, what if...

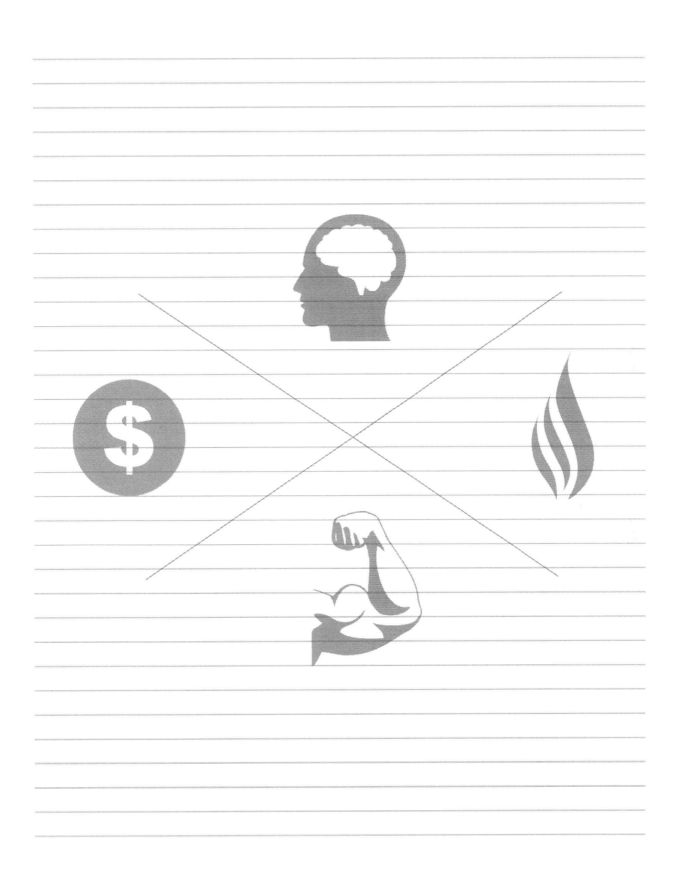

One sees great things from the valley; only small things from the peak. - G.K Chesterton

Date ___ / ___ / ___

Daily Priorities:

1 ....
....

2 ....
....

3 ....
....

4 ....
....

5 ....
....

6 ....
....

7 ....
....

8 ....
....

9 ....
....

Today I Appreciate:

1. _____

2. _____

3. _____

I'm strengthened knowing:

I'm looking forward to:

I will enrich my future by...

Mind ☐

☐ Meaning

Muscle ☐

☐ Money

With my health, what if...

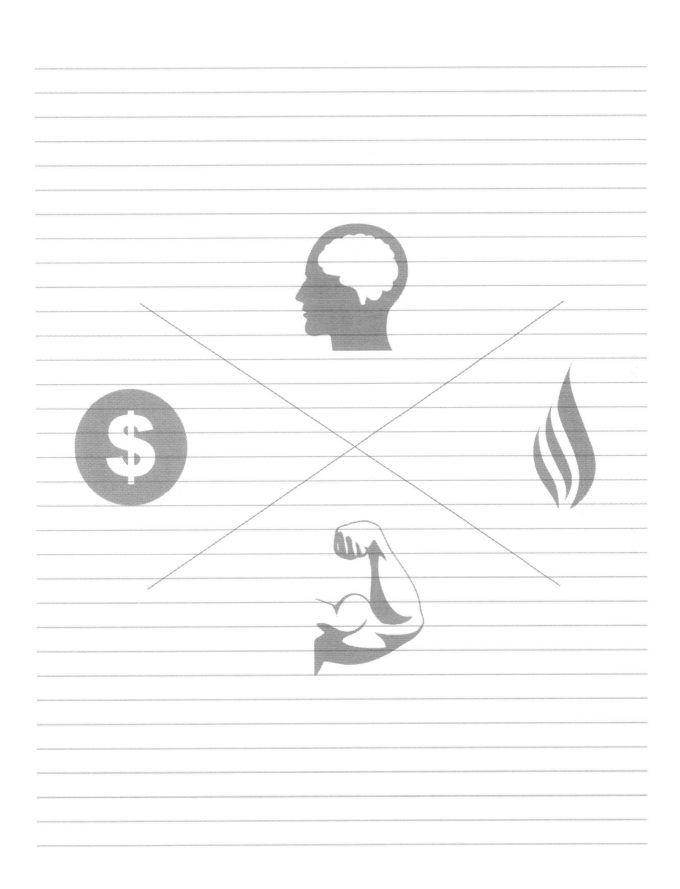

A business is a living, breathing organism. Neglect it, or allow toxicity to build up and it will wither and die.
Nurture and care for it and it will thrive and support all of its caregivers for life. - Mark Costes

Date _____ / _____ / _____

Today I Appreciate:

1. _____

2. _____

3. _____

Daily Priorities:

1

2

3

4

5

6

7

8

9

I'm strengthened knowing:

I'm looking forward to:

I will enrich my future by...

Mind ☐

☐ Meaning

Muscle ☐

☐ Money

With my daily spending habits, what if…

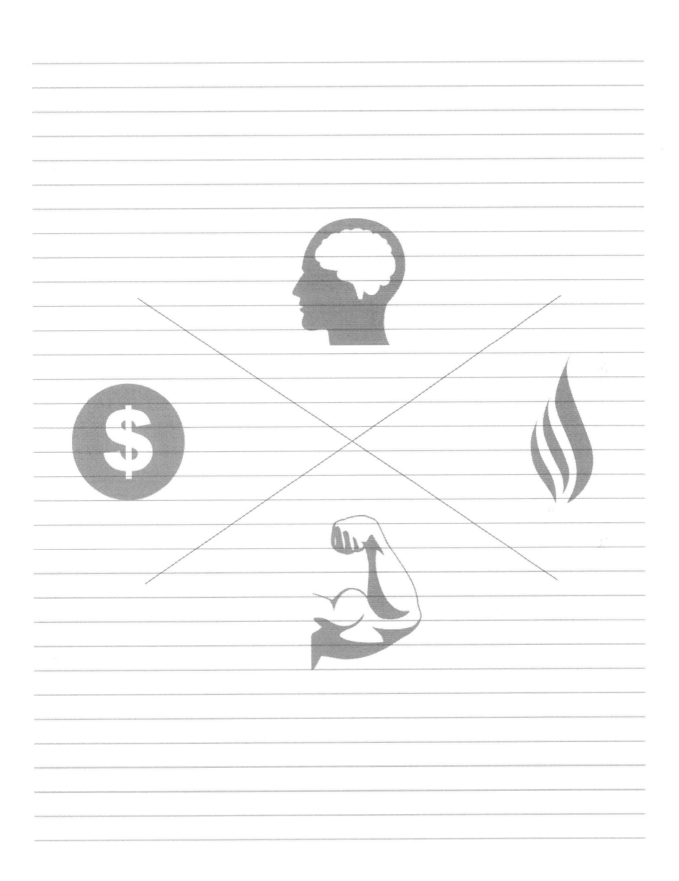

In the practice of tolerance, one's enemy is the best teacher. - Dalai Lama

Date ___ / ___ / ___

Daily Priorities:

1 ....
....
....

2 ....
....

3 ....
....

4 ....
....

5 ....
....

6 ....
....

7 ....
....

8 ....
....

9 ....
....

Today I Appreciate:

1. ....

2. ....

3. ....

I'm strengthened knowing:	I'm looking forward to:

I will enrich my future by...

Mind ☐   ☐ Meaning

Muscle ☐   ☐ Money

A bold move that I could make in order to improve my mind would be...

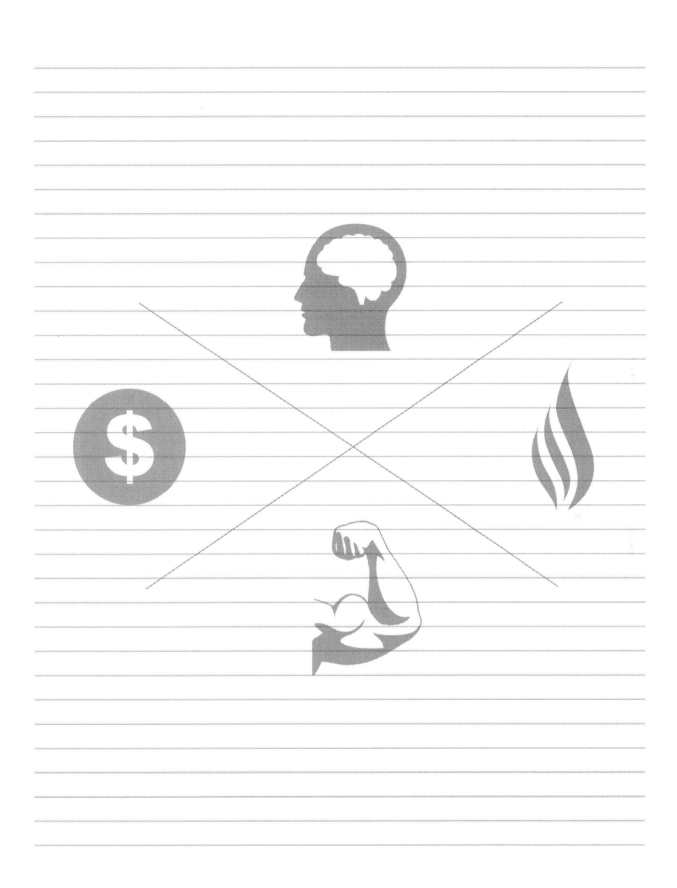

3 great things that happened this week:

_____

_____

_____

4 Futures Score Card

	M	T	W	R	F	S	S	Total	/28
Mind									/7
Meaning									/7
Muscle									/7
Money									/7

Next week, I will improve _____ by...	One area I excelled at this week

Looking Ahead to Next Week...

Major tasks I need to work on

My theme this week is...

Big events coming up that I need to prepare for:	I will improve my 4 Futures Score by doing the following:

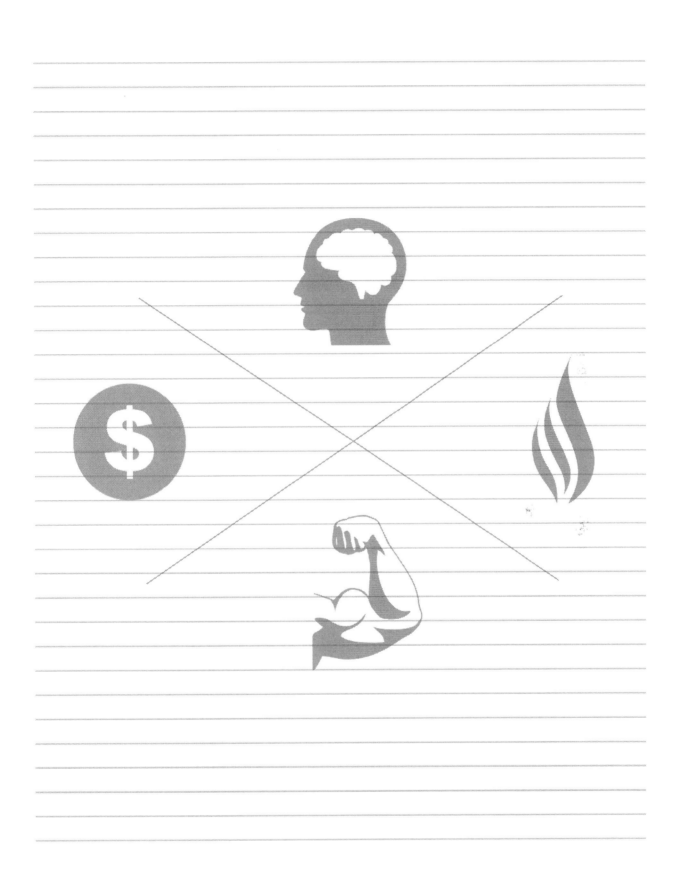

One doesn't discover new lands without consenting to lose sight of the shore for a very long time. - Andre Gide

Date ___/___/___

Daily Priorities:

1 ....

2 ....

3 ....

4 ....

5 ....

6 ....

7 ....

8 ....

9 ....

Today I Appreciate:

1. ....

2. ....

3. ....

I'm strengthened knowing:	I'm looking forward to:

I will enrich my future by...

Mind ☐   ☐ Meaning

Muscle ☐   ☐ Money

A bold move that I could make to improve meaning in my life would be:

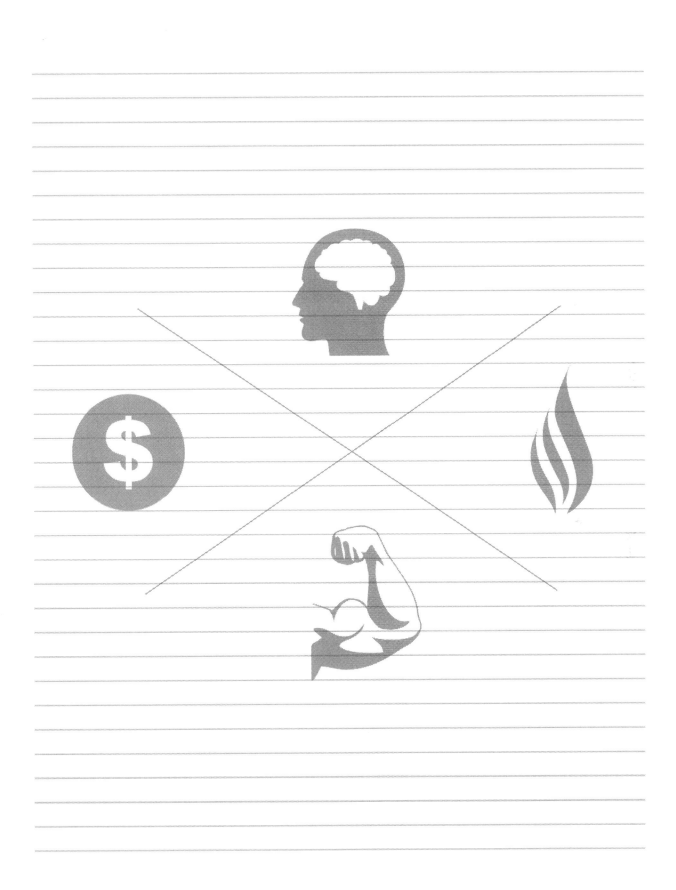

Peace is not absence of conflict, it is the ability to handle conflict by peaceful means. - Ronald Regan

Date ____ / ____ / ____

Daily Priorities:

1
2
3
4
5
6
7
8
9

Today I Appreciate:

1. _____
2. _____
3. _____

I'm strengthened knowing:

I'm looking forward to:

I will enrich my future by...

Mind ☐   ☐ Meaning

Muscle ☐   ☐ Money

A bold move that I could make in order to become more energetic would be:

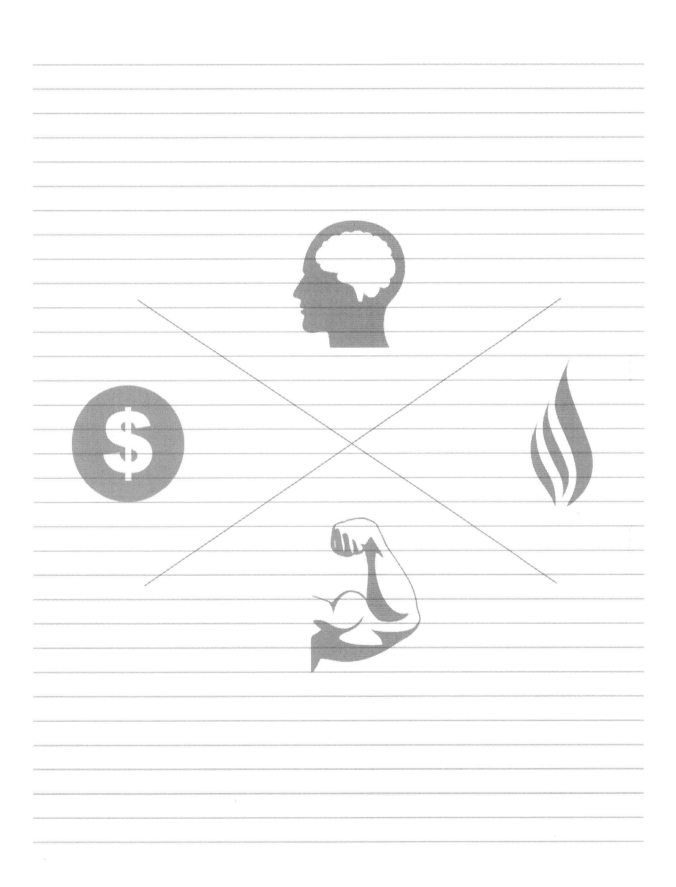

To learn who rules over you, simply find out who you are not allowed to criticize. - Voltaire

Date ___/___/___

Daily Priorities:

1
2
3
4
5
6
7
8
9

Today I Appreciate:
1. _____
2. _____
3. _____

I'm strengthened knowing:

I'm looking forward to:

I will enrich my future by...

Mind ☐   ☐ Meaning

Muscle ☐   ☐ Money

A bold move that I could make financially would be:

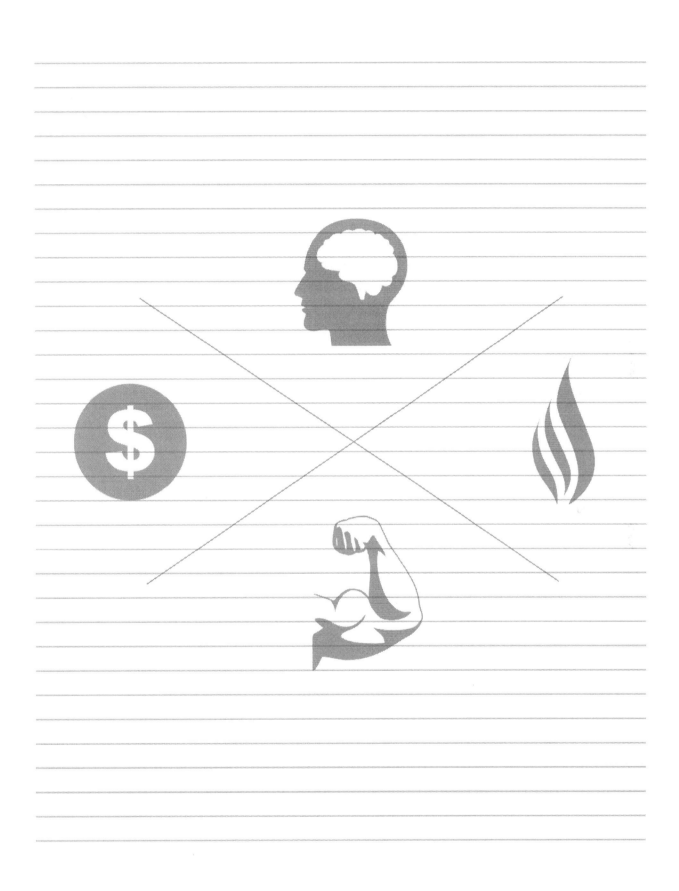

Date _____ / _____ / _____

Today I Appreciate:

1. _____
2. _____
3. _____

Daily Priorities:

1 ....

2 ....

3 ....

4 ....

5 ....

6 ....

7 ....

8 ....

9 ....

I'm strengthened knowing:

I'm looking forward to:

I will enrich my future by...

Mind ☐

☐ Meaning

Muscle ☐

☐ Money

A concept worth investigating in order to improve feelings of stress...

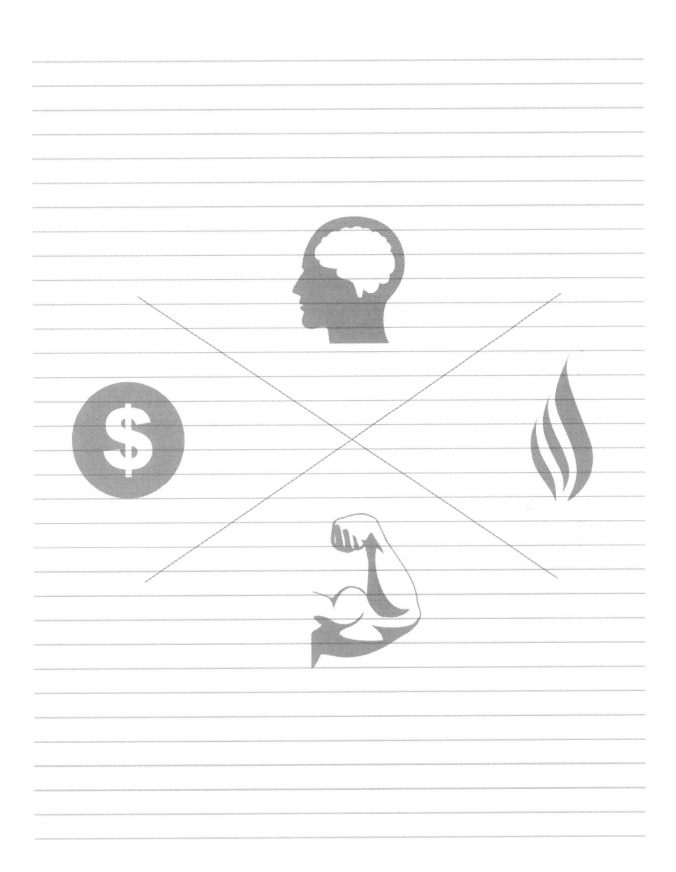

Date ____ / ____ / ____

Daily Priorities:

1

2

3

4

5

6

7

8

9

Today I Appreciate:

1. _____

2. _____

3. _____

I'm strengthened knowing:

I'm looking forward to:

I will enrich my future by...

Mind ☐

☐ Meaning

Muscle ☐

☐ Money

A concept worth investigating in order to improve the relationships of those who mean the most to me would be:

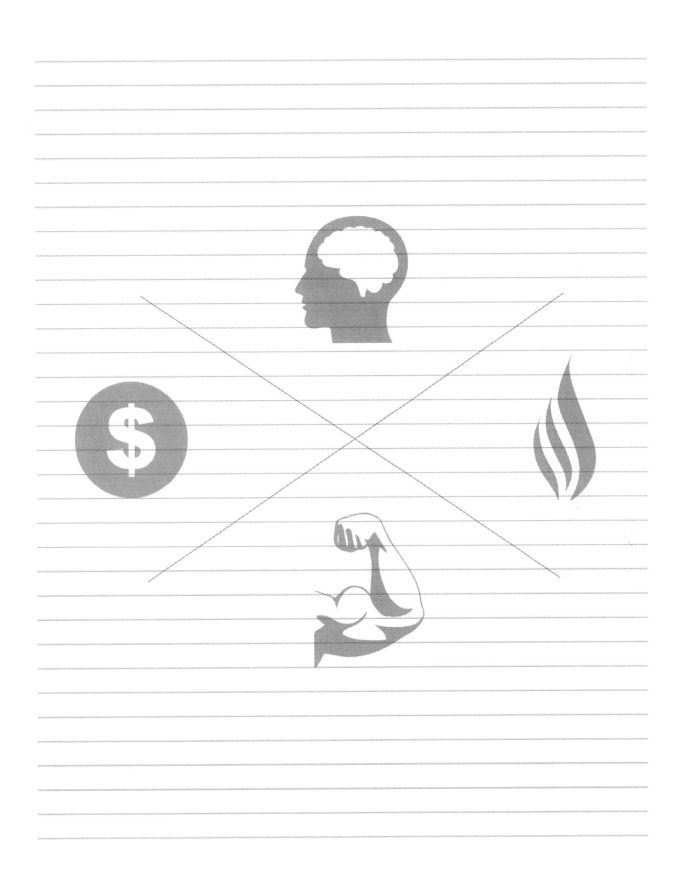

Date _____ / _____ / _____

Daily Priorities:

1 ....
....
....

2 ....
....

3 ....
....

4 ....
....

5 ....
....

6 ....
....

7 ....
....

8 ....
....

9 ....
....

Today I Appreciate:

1. _____

2. _____

3. _____

I'm strengthened knowing:	I'm looking forward to:

I will enrich my future by...

Mind ☐   ☐ Meaning

Muscle ☐   ☐ Money

A concept worth investigating in order to improve my health would be:

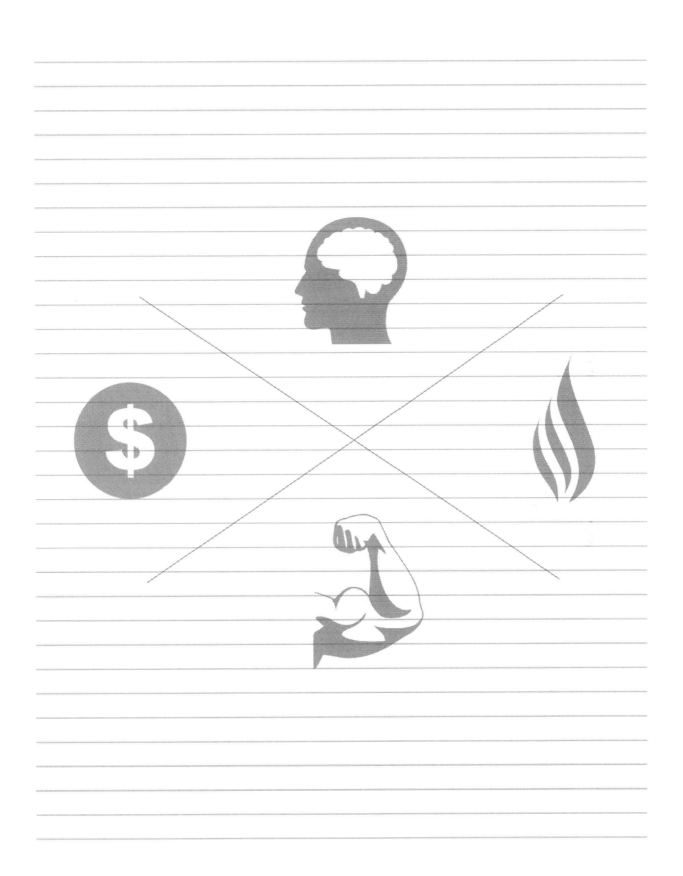

Date _____ / _____ / _____

Today I Appreciate:

1. _____

2. _____

3. _____

Daily Priorities:

1 ....

2 ....

3 ....

4 ....

5 ....

6 ....

7 ....

8 ....

9 ....

I'm strengthened knowing:

I'm looking forward to:

I will enrich my future by...

Mind ☐

☐ Meaning

Muscle ☐

☐ Money

A concept worth investigating in order to reduce financial stress would be:

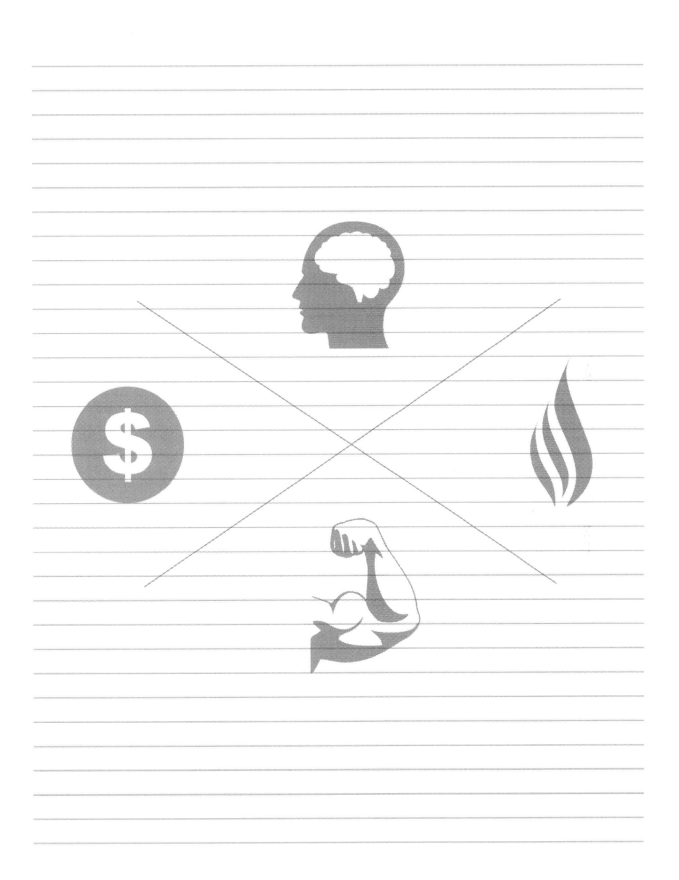

Weekly Wrap-Up

3 great things that happened this week:

_____

_____

_____

4 Futures Score Card

	M	T	W	R	F	S	S	Total	/28
Mind									/7
Meaning									/7
Muscle									/7
Money									/7

Next week, I will improve _____ by...	One area I excelled at this week

Looking Ahead to Next Week...

Major tasks I need to work on

My theme this week is...

Big events coming up that I need to prepare for:	I will improve my 4 Futures Score by doing the following:

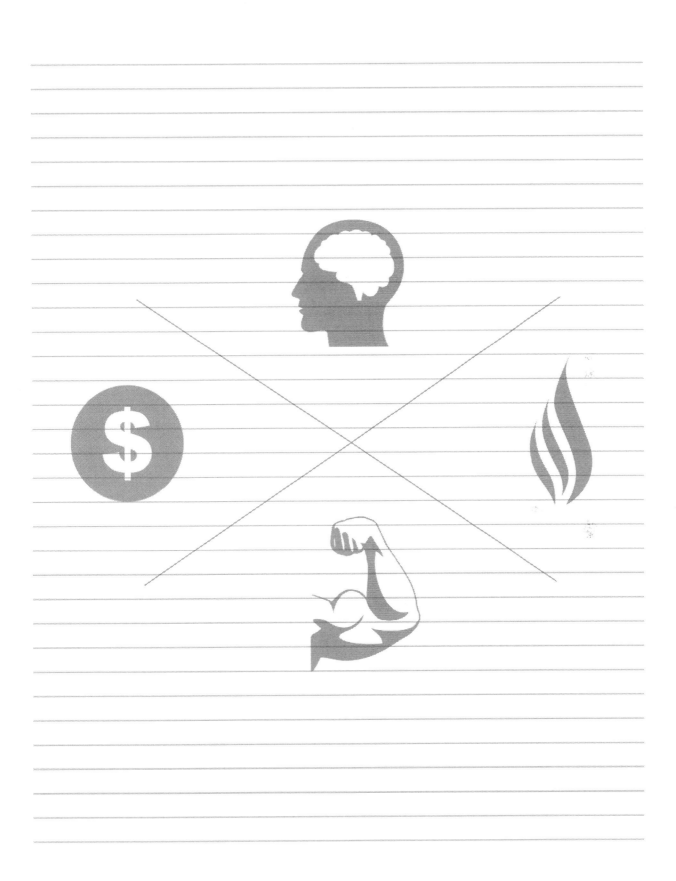

Because things are the way they are, things will not stay the way they are. - Bertolt Brecht

Date ___ / ___ / ___

Daily Priorities:

1 ....
....
....

2 ....
....

3 ....
....

4 ....
....

5 ....
....

6 ....
....

7 ....
....

8 ....
....

9 ....
....

Today I Appreciate:

1. _____

2. _____

3. _____

I'm strengthened knowing:

I'm looking forward to:

I will enrich my future by...

Mind ☐

☐ Meaning

Muscle ☐

☐ Money

A common theme I'm seeing in my thought patterns...

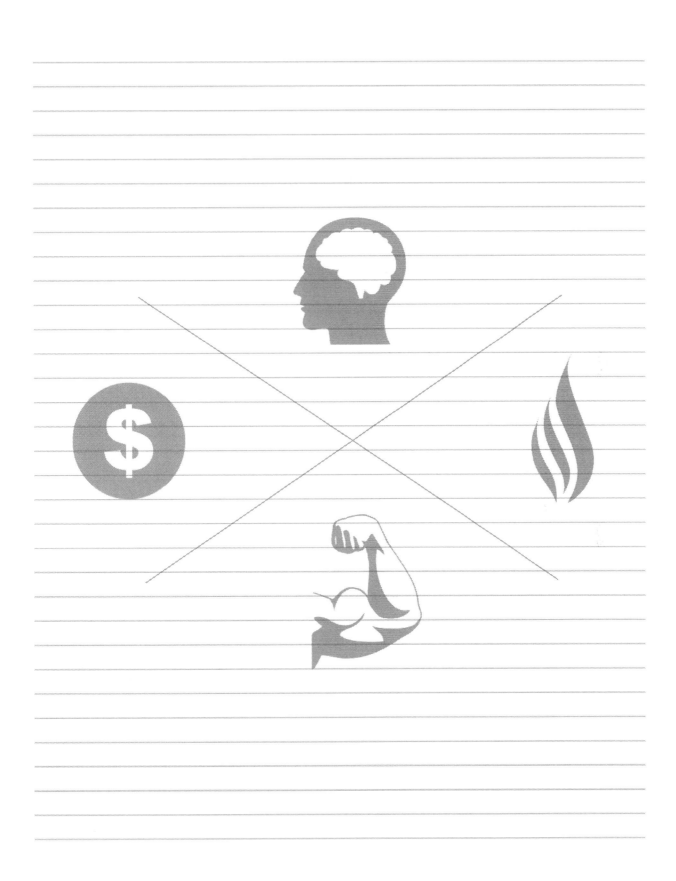

Date ___ / ___ / ___

Daily Priorities:

1
2
3
4
5
6
7
8
9

Today I Appreciate:

1. ....

2. ....

3. ....

I'm strengthened knowing:	I'm looking forward to:

I will enrich my future by...

Mind ☐   ☐ Meaning

Muscle ☐   ☐ Money

A common theme that I'm seeing in my relationships…

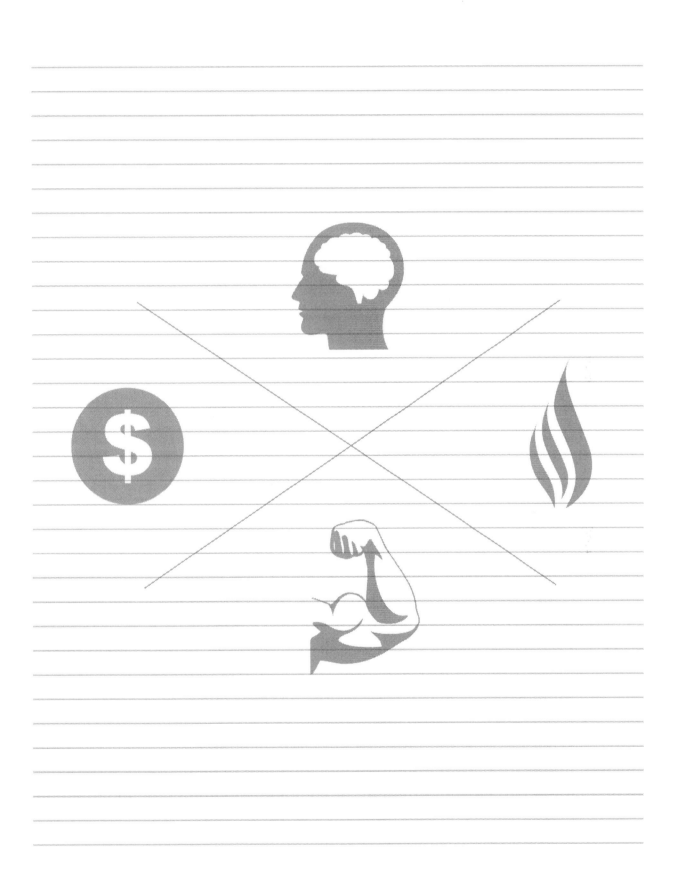

Hunger is the best sauce in the world. - Miguel de Cervantes Saavedra

Date _____ / _____ / _____

Today I Appreciate:

1. _____
2. _____
3. _____

Daily Priorities:

1
2
3
4
5
6
7
8
9

I'm strengthened knowing:

I'm looking forward to:

I will enrich my future by...

Mind ☐   ☐ Meaning

Muscle ☐   ☐ Money

A common theme that I'm seeing in my health...

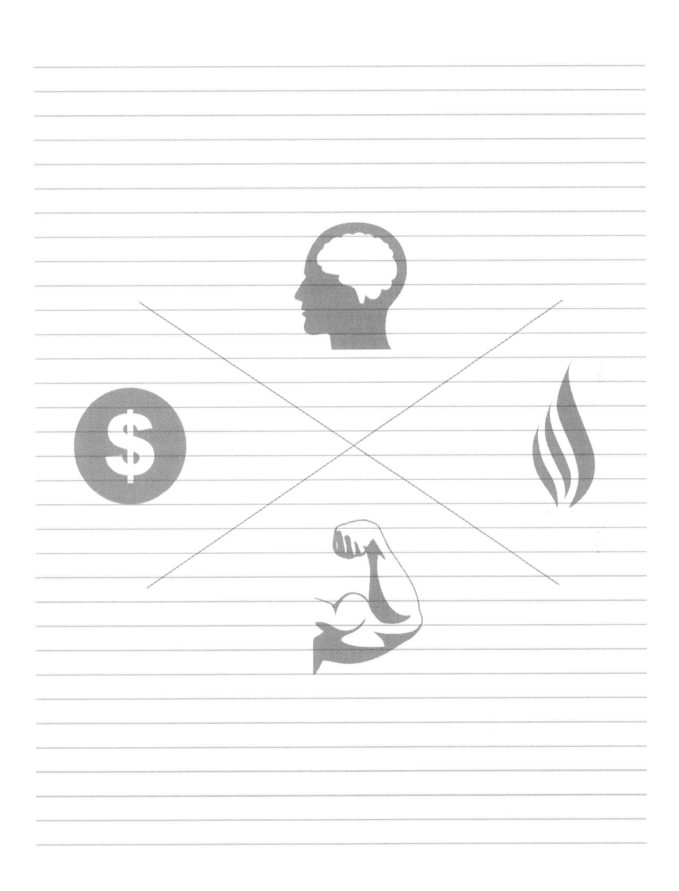

Changing trajectory by one degree is a powerful tool - Since that change, done early,
can land you on a completely different planet. - Mark Costes

Date _____ / _____ / _____

Daily Priorities:

1
2
3
4
5
6
7
8
9

Today I Appreciate:

1. _____

2. _____

3. _____

I'm strengthened knowing:

I'm looking forward to:

I will enrich my future by...

Mind ☐   ☐ Meaning

Muscle ☐   ☐ Money

A common financial theme that I'm seeing...

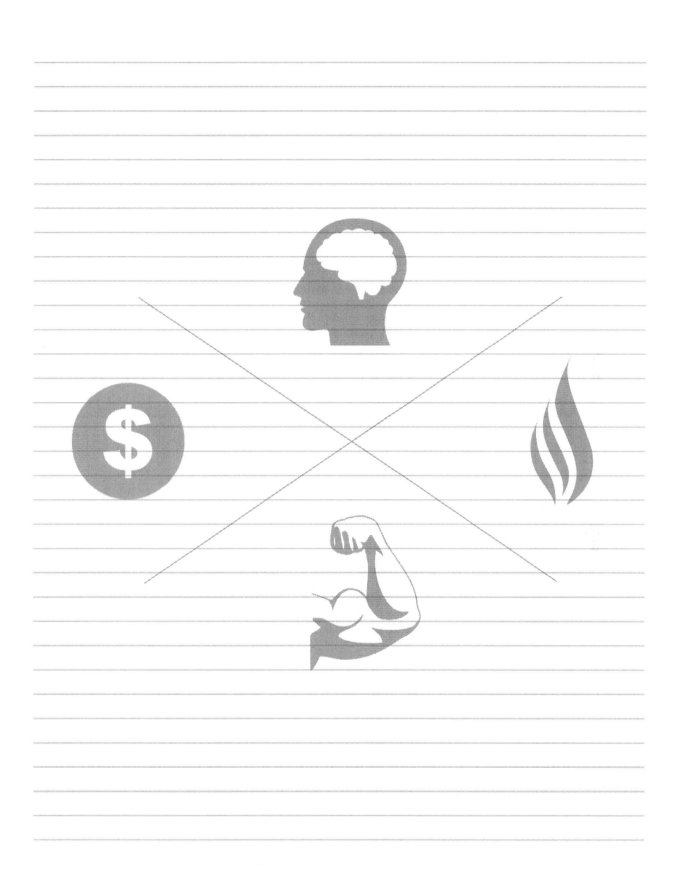

I will not let anyone walk through my mind with their dirty feet. - Mahatma Gandhi

Date _____ / _____ / _____

Daily Priorities:

1 ....
....

2 ....
....

3 ....
....

4 ....
....

5 ....
....

6 ....
....

7 ....
....

8 ....
....

9 ....
....

Today I Appreciate:

1. _____

2. _____

3. _____

I'm strengthened knowing:

I'm looking forward to:

I will enrich my future by...

Mind ☐   ☐ Meaning

Muscle ☐   ☐ Money

Something for me to contemplate with my self control is...

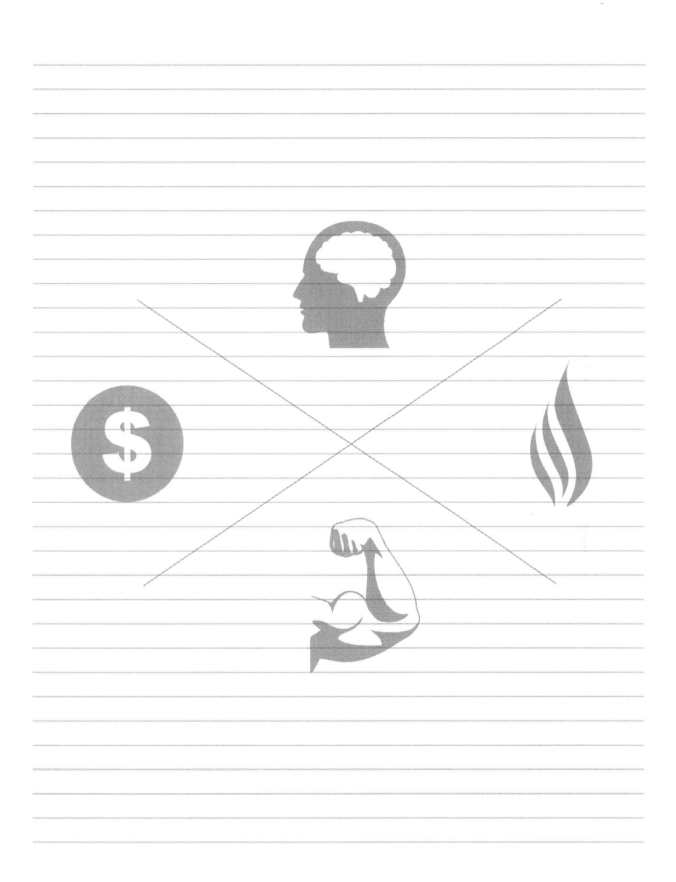

Date _____ / _____ / _____

Daily Priorities:

1

2

3

4

5

6

7

8

9

Today I Appreciate:

1. _____

2. _____

3. _____

I'm strengthened knowing:

I'm looking forward to:

I will enrich my future by...

Mind ☐

☐ Meaning

Muscle ☐

☐ Money

Something for me to contemplate in my relationships...

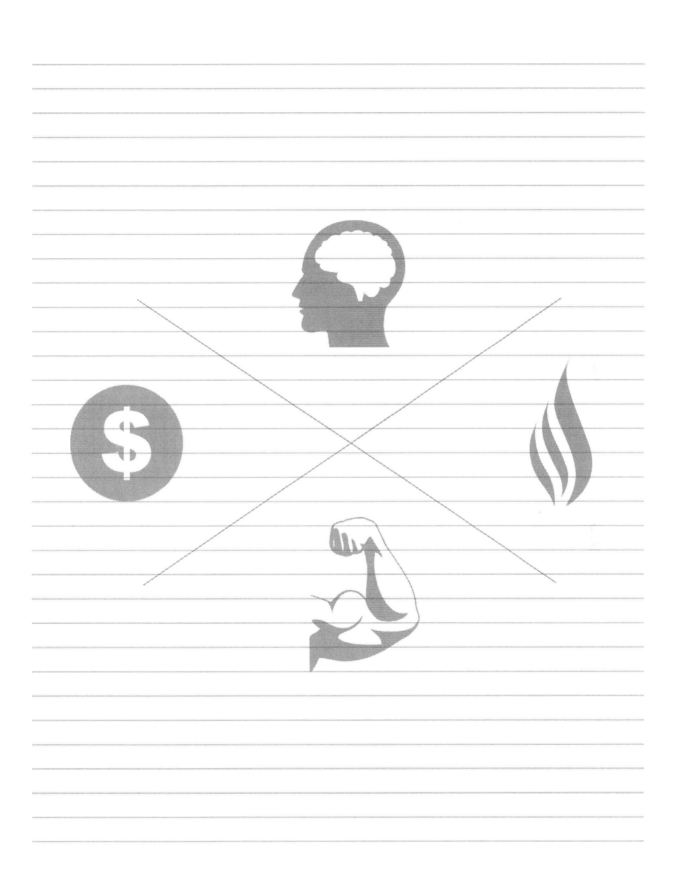

The wounds recieved in battle bestow honor, they do not take it away. - Miguel de Cervantes Saavedra

Date ____ / ____ / ____

Daily Priorities:

1

2

3

4

5

6

7

8

9

Today I Appreciate:

1. _____

2. _____

3. _____

I'm strengthened knowing:

I'm looking forward to:

I will enrich my future by...

Mind ☐

☐ Meaning

Muscle ☐

☐ Money

Something for me to contemplate to improve how I feel physically...

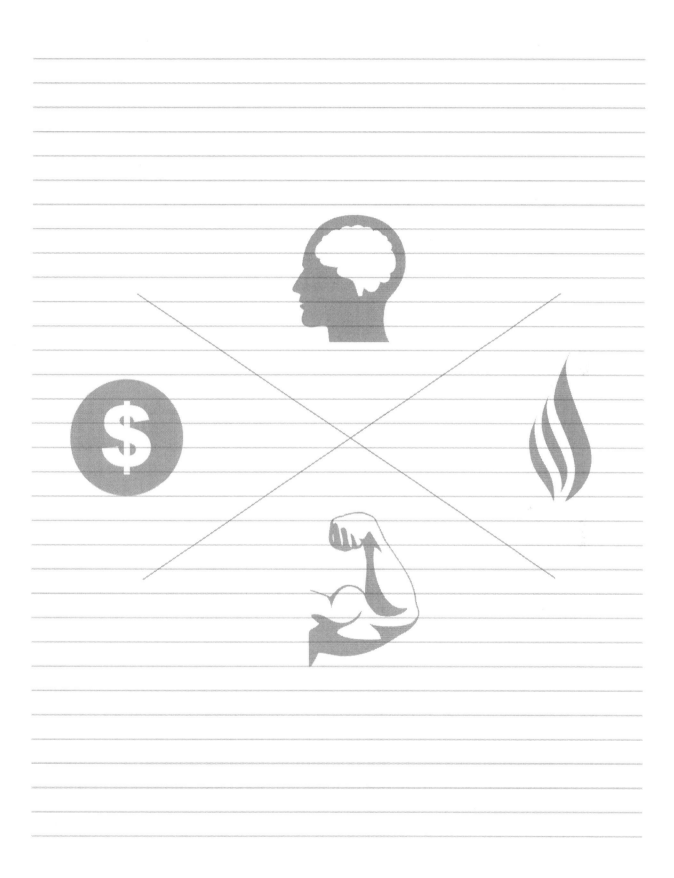

Weekly Wrap-Up

3 great things that happened this week:

_____

_____

_____

4 Futures Score Card

	M	T	W	R	F	S	S	Total	/28
Mind									/7
Meaning									/7
Muscle									/7
Money									/7

Next week, I will improve _____ by...	One area I excelled at this week

Looking Ahead to Next Week...

Major tasks I need to work on

My theme this week is...

Big events coming up that I need to prepare for:	I will improve my 4 Futures Score by doing the following:

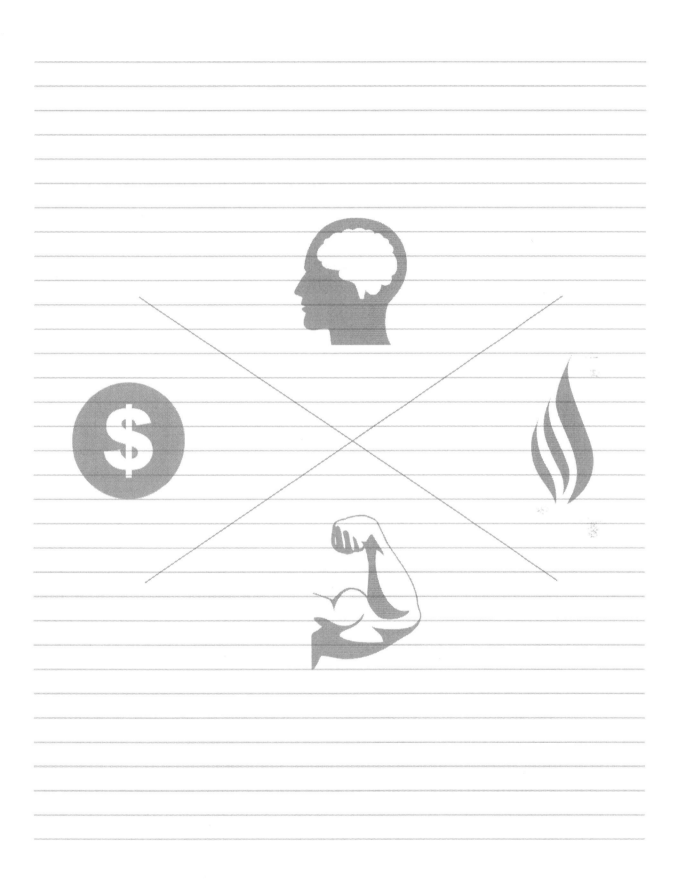

Date   /   /

Daily Priorities:

1
2
3
4
5
6
7
8
9

Today I Appreciate:

1. _____

2. _____

3. _____

I'm strengthened knowing:

I'm looking forward to:

I will enrich my future by...

Mind ☐

☐ Meaning

Muscle ☐

☐ Money

Something for me to contemplate in order to improve my long-term financial safety...

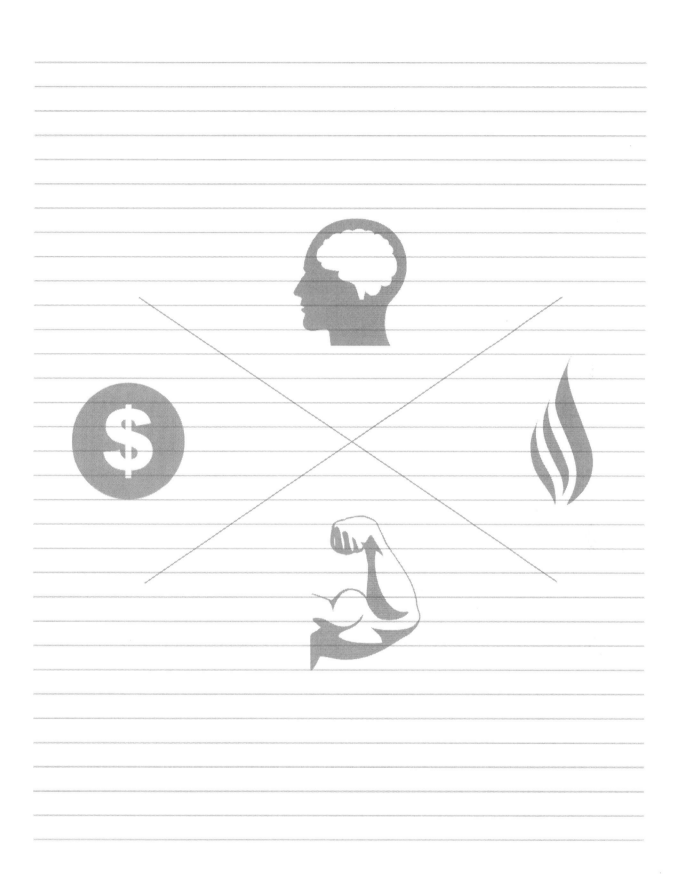

Nothing is so firmly believed as that which we least know. - Michel de Montaigne

Date ___ / ___ / ___

Daily Priorities:

1
2
3
4
5
6
7
8
9

Today I Appreciate:

1. _____
2. _____
3. _____

I'm strengthened knowing:

I'm looking forward to:

I will enrich my future by...

Mind ☐

☐ Meaning

Muscle ☐

☐ Money

With my mental focus, what if…

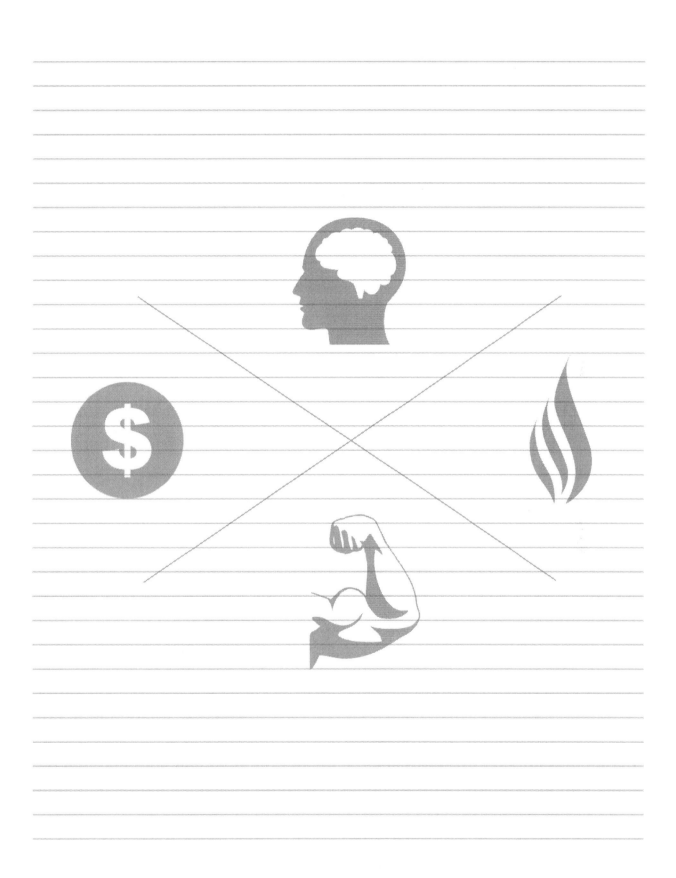

*You can get as much guidance from paying attention to the behaviors of your anti-heroes
as you can from modeling your heroes. - Mark Costes*

Date ___ / ___ / ___

Daily Priorities:

1
2
3
4
5
6
7
8
9

Today I Appreciate:

1. _____
2. _____
3. _____

I'm strengthened knowing:

I'm looking forward to:

I will enrich my future by...

Mind ☐

☐ Meaning

Muscle ☐

☐ Money

To become closer to those around me, What if…

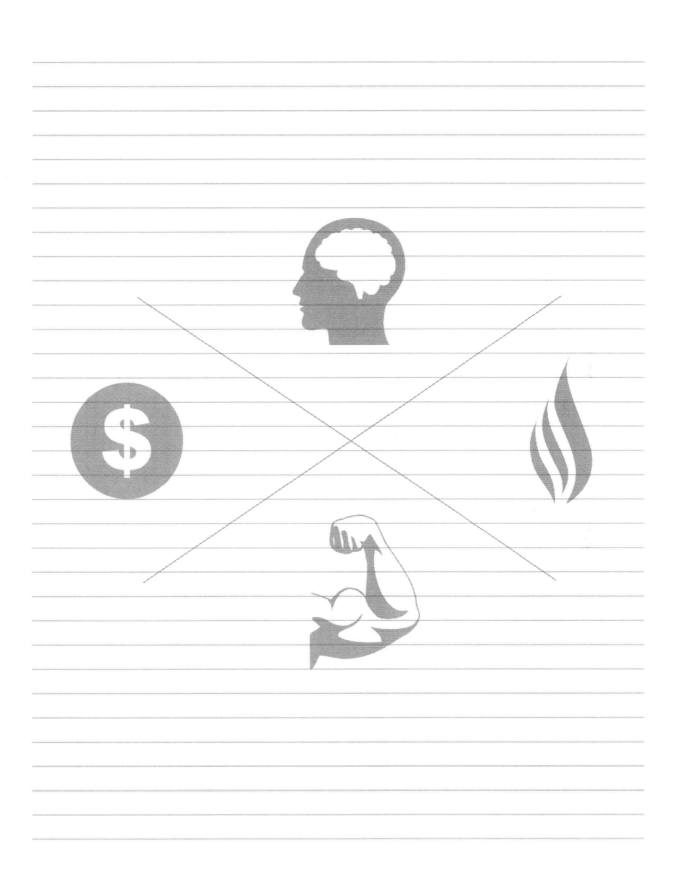

Date _____ / _____ / _____

Daily Priorities:

1 ....
....
2 ....
....
3 ....
....
4 ....
....
5 ....
....
6 ....
....
7 ....
....
8 ....
....
9 ....
....

Today I Appreciate:

1. _____

2. _____

3. _____

I'm strengthened knowing:

I'm looking forward to:

I will enrich my future by...

Mind ☐

☐ Meaning

Muscle ☐

☐ Money

With my health, What if...

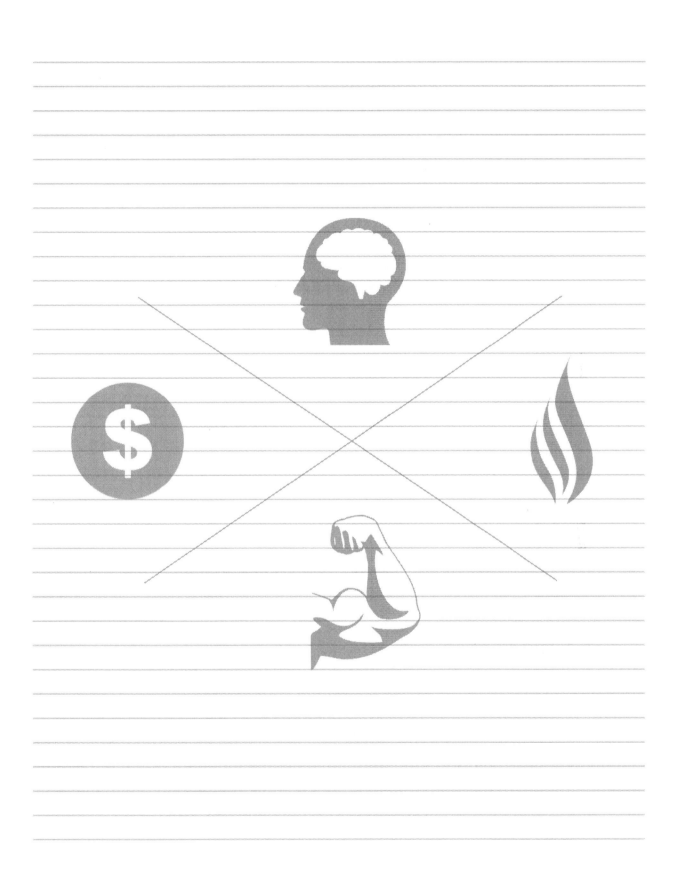

Date ___ / ___ / ___

Today I Appreciate:

1. _____

2. _____

3. _____

Daily Priorities:

1

2

3

4

5

6

7

8

9

I'm strengthened knowing:

I'm looking forward to:

I will enrich my future by...

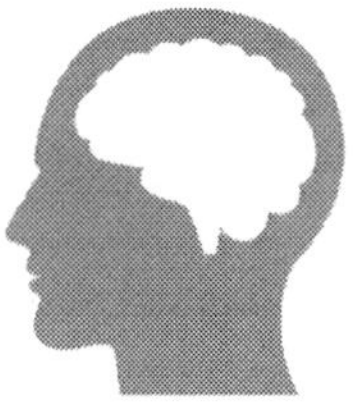

Mind ☐

☐ Meaning

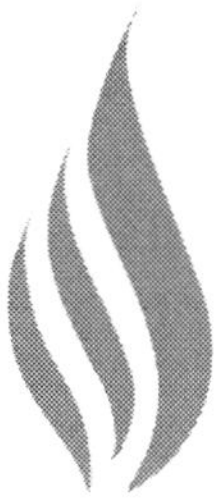

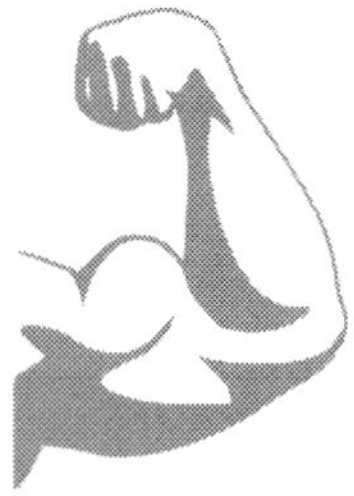

Muscle ☐

☐ Money

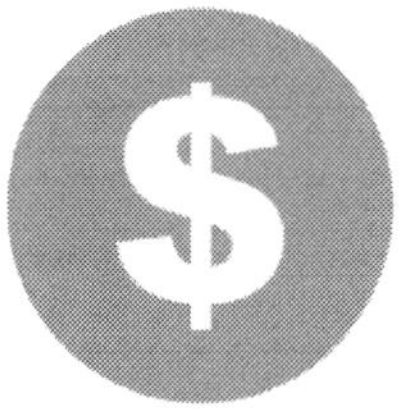

With my daily spending habits, What if...

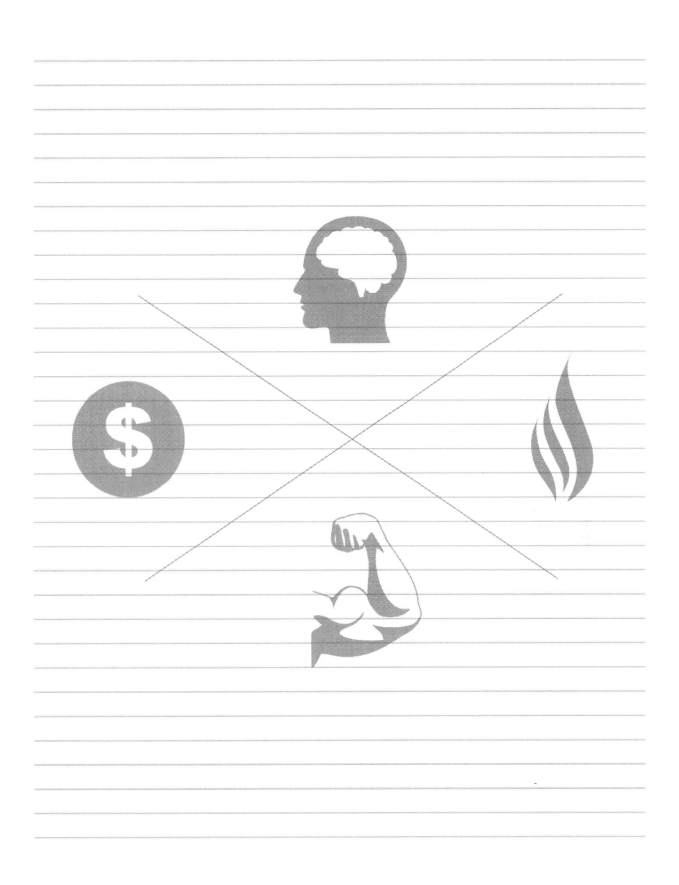

Of all the influences that effect change, boredom may be the most powerful.
Own it and design the change, or ignore it and it will change you. - Alastair Macdonald

Date _____ / _____ / _____

Today I Appreciate:

1. _____

2. _____

3. _____

Daily Priorities:

1 ....

2 ....

3 ....

4 ....

5 ....

6 ....

7 ....

8 ....

9 ....

I'm strengthened knowing:

I'm looking forward to:

I will enrich my future by...

Mind ☐

☐ Meaning

Muscle ☐

☐ Money

A bold move that I could make to improve my mind would be:

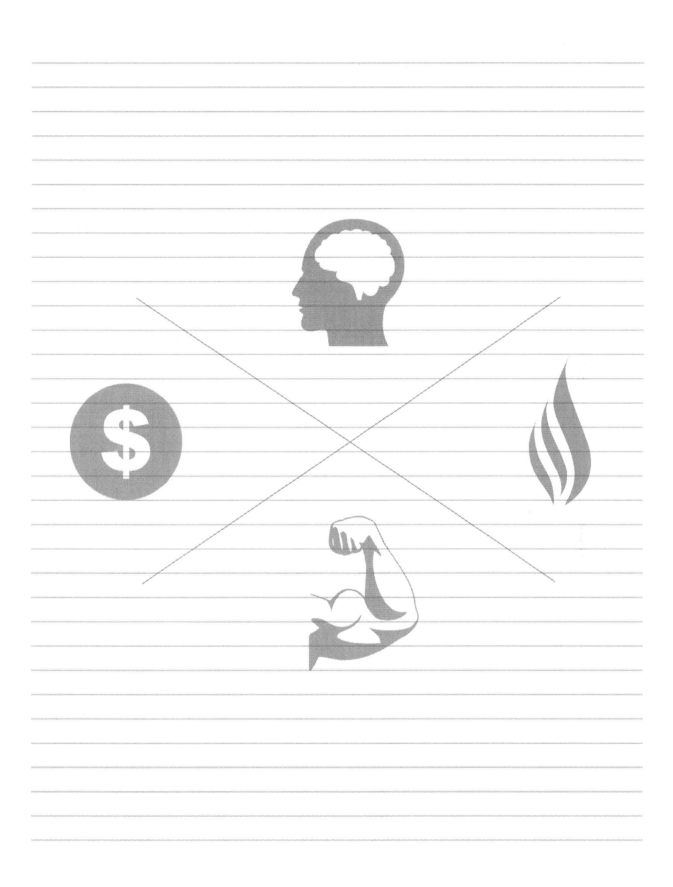

I want to age and die through archiving my experiences, not watching my biological clock. Please don't waste my clock time with mediocrity and egotism, let me use it towards serving to others. - Alper Mazun

Date _____ / _____ / _____

Today I Appreciate:

1. _____
2. _____
3. _____

Daily Priorities:

1

2

3

4

5

6

7

8

9

I'm strengthened knowing:

I'm looking forward to:

I will enrich my future by...

Mind ☐   ☐ Meaning

Muscle ☐   ☐ Money

A bold move that I could make to improve meaning in my life would be:

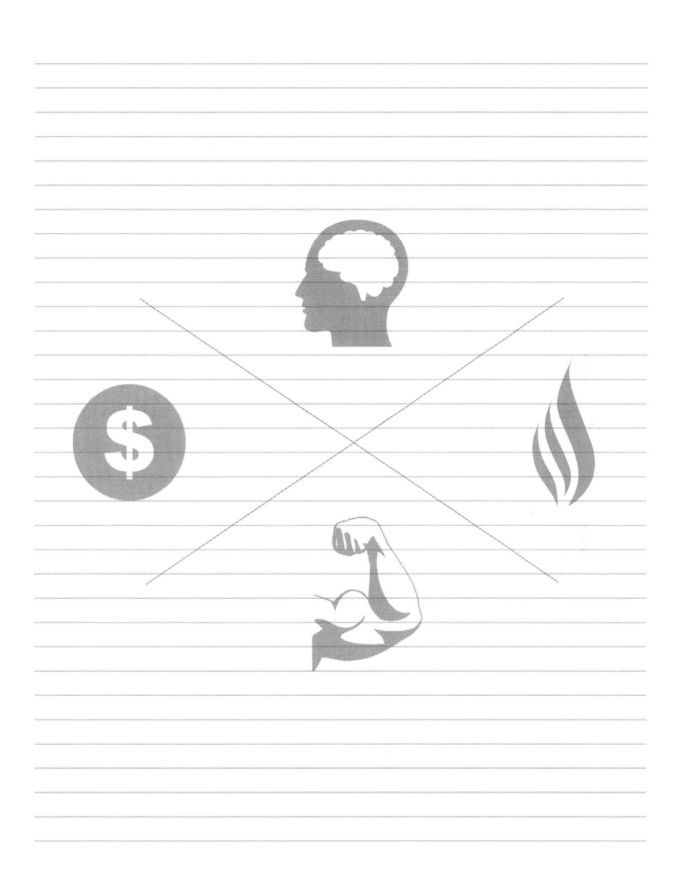

Weekly Wrap-Up

3 great things that happened this week:

....

....

....

4 Futures Score Card

	M	T	W	R	F	S	S	Total	/28
Mind									/7
Meaning									/7
Muscle									/7
Money									/7

Next week, I will improve _____ by...	One area I excelled at this week

Looking Ahead to Next Week...

Major tasks I need to work on

My theme this week is...

Big events coming up that I need to prepare for:	I will improve my 4 Futures Score by doing the following:

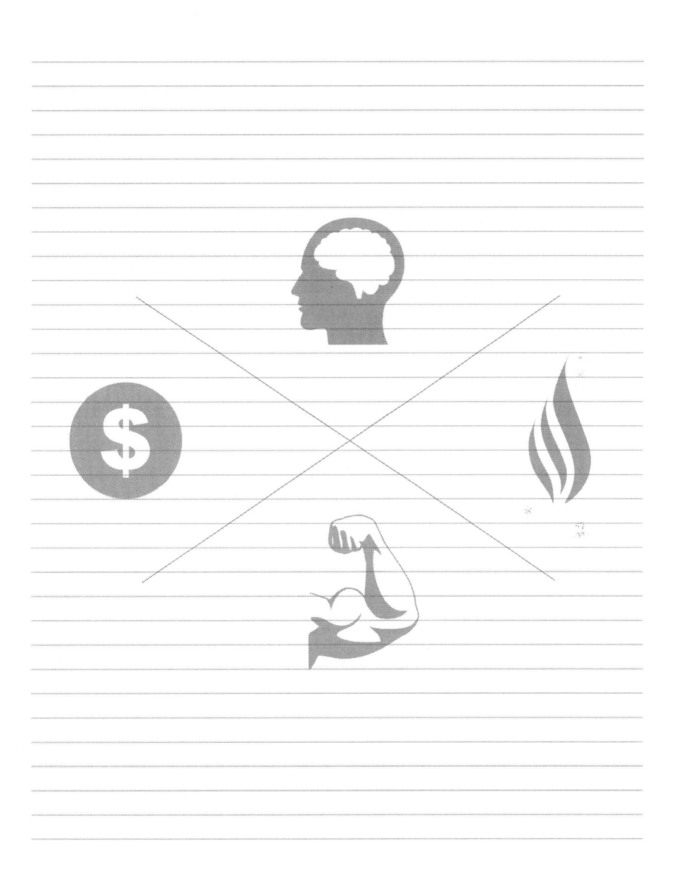

I know the day I start giving in to my fears in one area of my life, it will only be a matter of time before it becomes easier to avoid other challenges as well. - Andrea Waltz

Date _____ / _____ / _____

Daily Priorities:

1
2
3
4
5
6
7
8
9

Today I Appreciate:

1. _____
2. _____
3. _____

I'm strengthened knowing:

I'm looking forward to:

I will enrich my future by...

Mind ☐

☐ Meaning

Muscle ☐

☐ Money

A bold move that I could make to become more energetic would be:

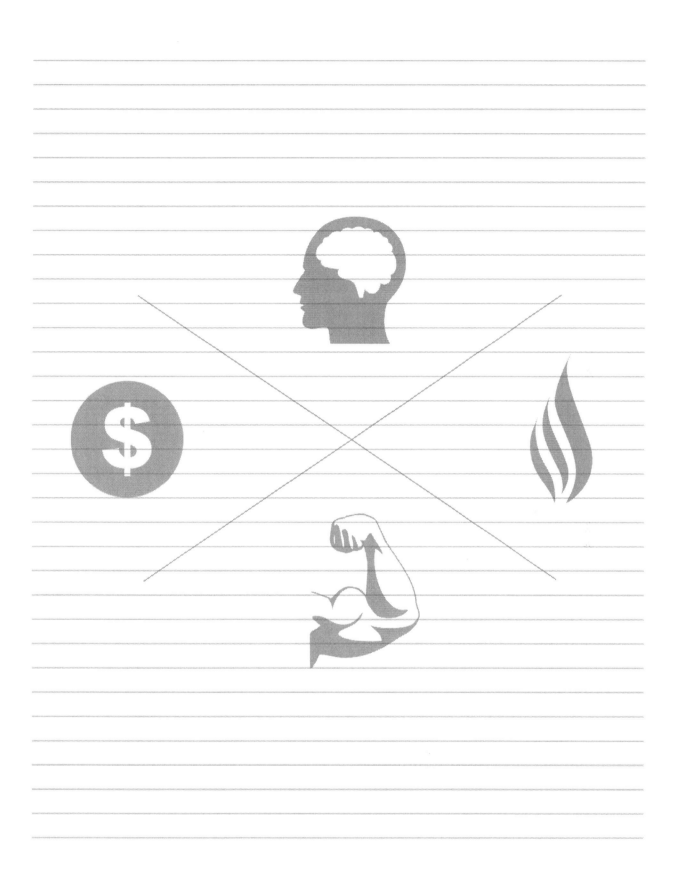

Date ___ / ___ / ___

Today I Appreciate:

1. _____

2. _____

3. _____

Daily Priorities:

1

2

3

4

5

6

7

8

9

I'm strengthened knowing:

I'm looking forward to:

I will enrich my future by...

Mind ☐

☐ Meaning

Muscle ☐

☐ Money

A bold move that I could make financially would be:

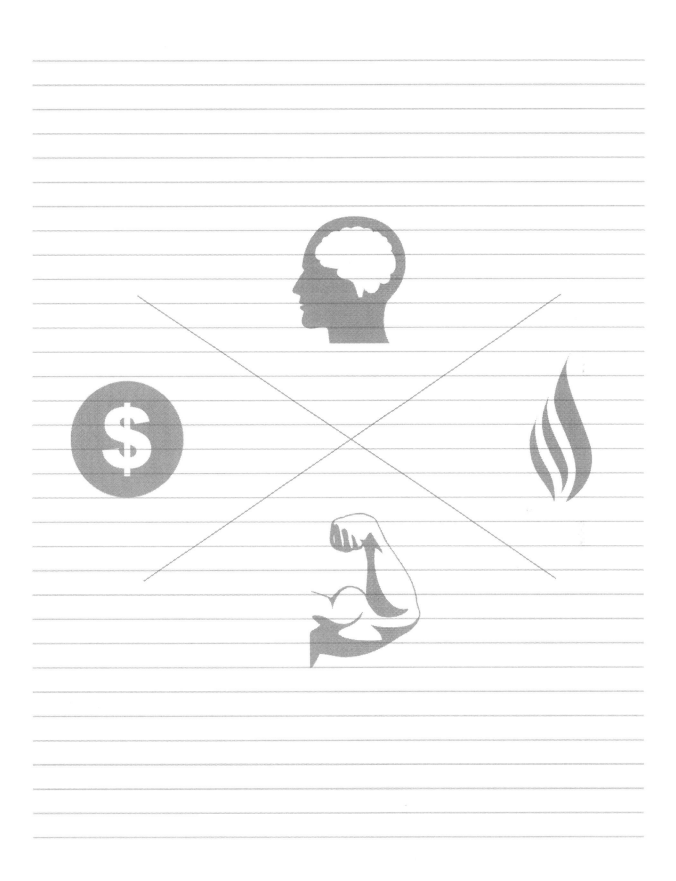

*It is not the strongest of the species that survives, nor the most intelligent,
but rather the one most adaptable to change. - Clarence Darrow*

Date _____ / _____ / _____

Daily Priorities:

1 ....
....

2 ....
....

3 ....
....

4 ....
....

5 ....
....

6 ....
....

7 ....
....

8 ....
....

9 ....
....

Today I Appreciate:

1. ....

2. ....

3. ....

I'm strengthened knowing:

I'm looking forward to:

I will enrich my future by...

Mind ☐

☐ Meaning

Muscle ☐

☐ Money

A concept worth investigating to improve feelings of stress…

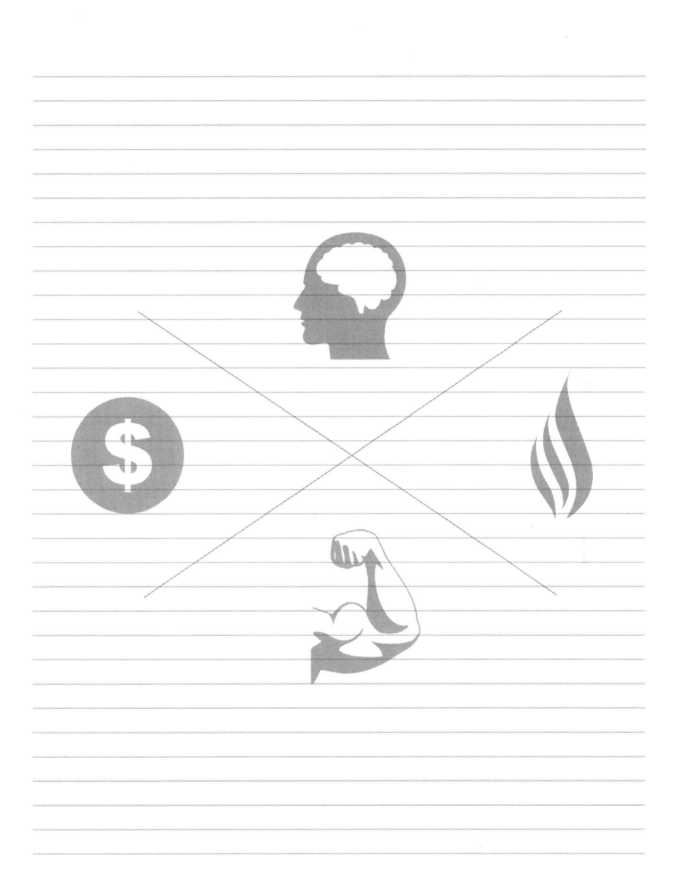

Date _____ / _____ / _____

Daily Priorities:

1 ....
....

2 ....
....

3 ....
....

4 ....
....

5 ....
....

6 ....
....

7 ....
....

8 ....
....

9 ....
....

Today I Appreciate:

1. _____

2. _____

3. _____

I'm strengthened knowing:

I'm looking forward to:

I will enrich my future by...

Mind ☐   ☐ Meaning

Muscle ☐   ☐ Money

A concept worth investigating to improve the relationships of those who mean the most to me would be:

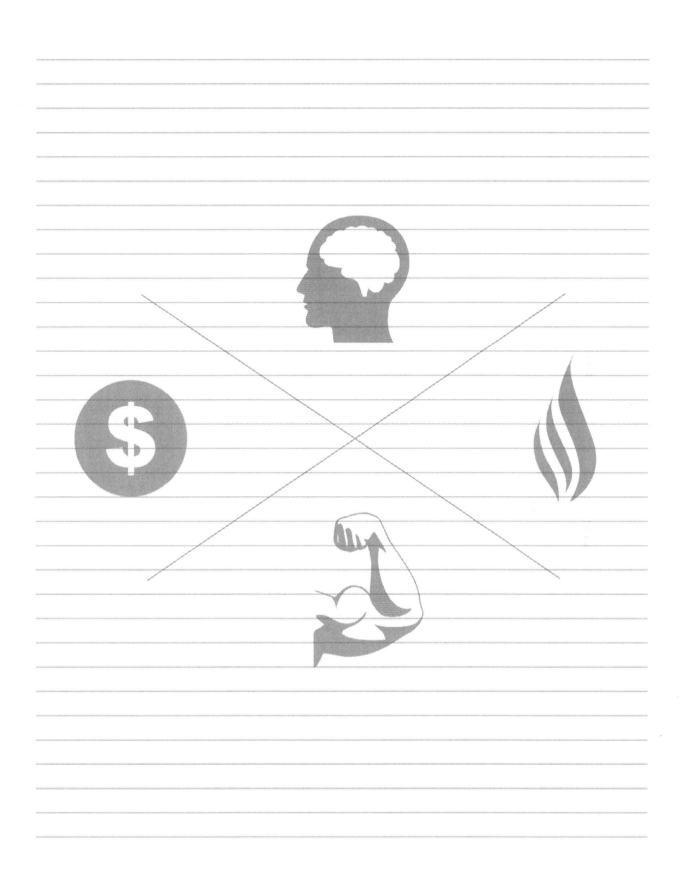

Many men go fishing all of their lives without knowing that it is not fish they are after. - Henry David Thoreau

Date _____ / _____ / _____

Daily Priorities:

1
2
3
4
5
6
7
8
9

Today I Appreciate:

1. _____

2. _____

3. _____

I'm strengthened knowing:

I'm looking forward to:

I will enrich my future by...

Mind ☐   ☐ Meaning

Muscle ☐   ☐ Money

A concept worth investigating to improve my health:

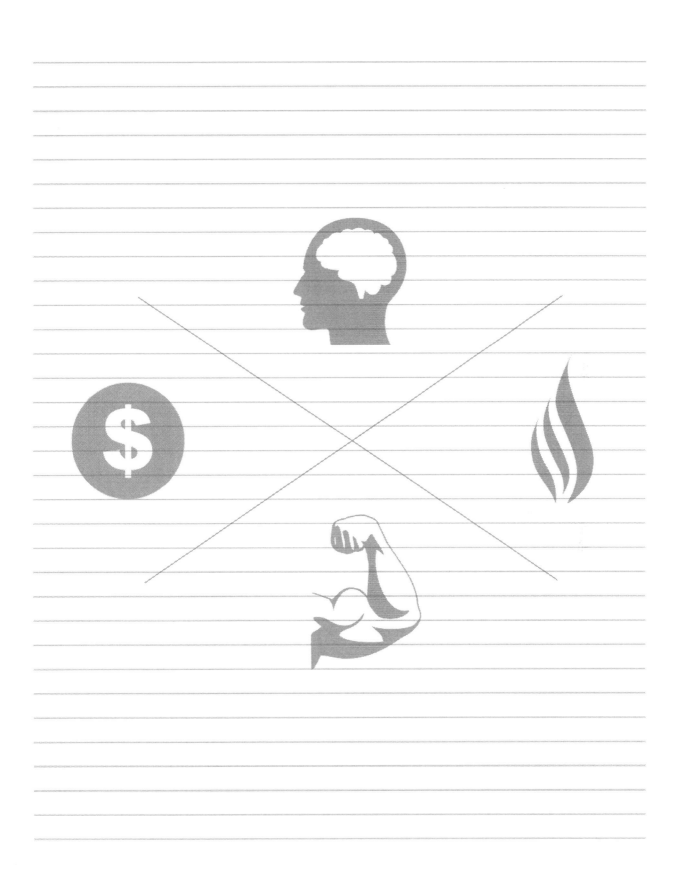

Date _____ / _____ / _____

Today I Appreciate:

1. ....

2. ....

3. ....

Daily Priorities:

1

2

3

4

5

6

7

8

9

I'm strengthened knowing:

I'm looking forward to:

I will enrich my future by...

Mind ☐

☐ Meaning

Muscle ☐

☐ Money

A concept worth investigating in order to reduce financial stress would be:

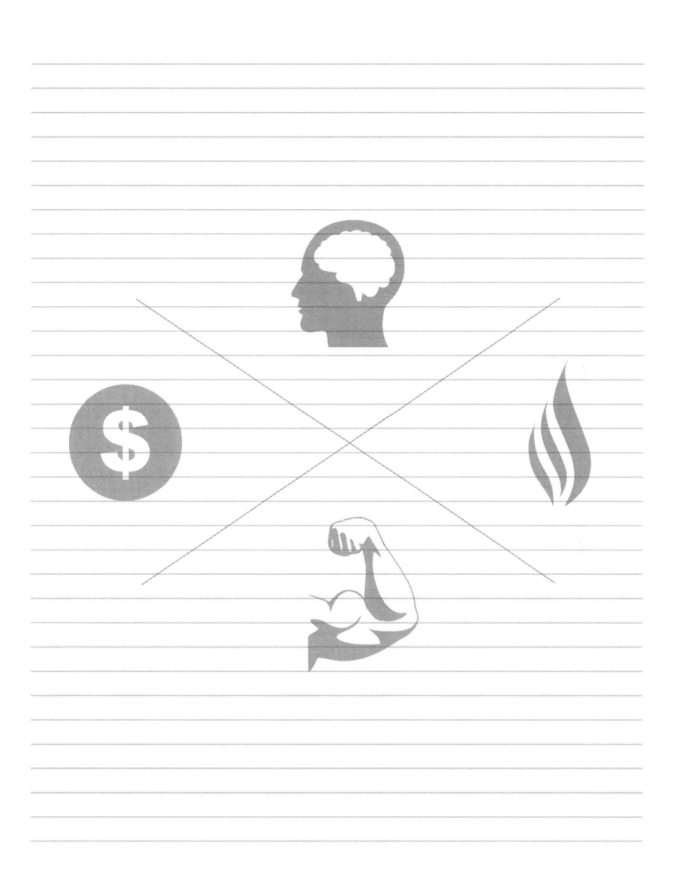

There is no physiologic effect larger than the Placebo effect. - Mathew Walker PhD

Date _____ / _____ / _____

Daily Priorities:

1 ....
....

2 ....
....

3 ....
....

4 ....
....

5 ....
....

6 ....
....

7 ....
....

8 ....
....

9 ....
....

Today I Appreciate:

1. _____

2. _____

3. _____

I'm strengthened knowing:

I'm looking forward to:

I will enrich my future by...

Mind ☐

☐ Meaning

Muscle ☐

☐ Money

Sometimes I let these thoughts overpower my mind:

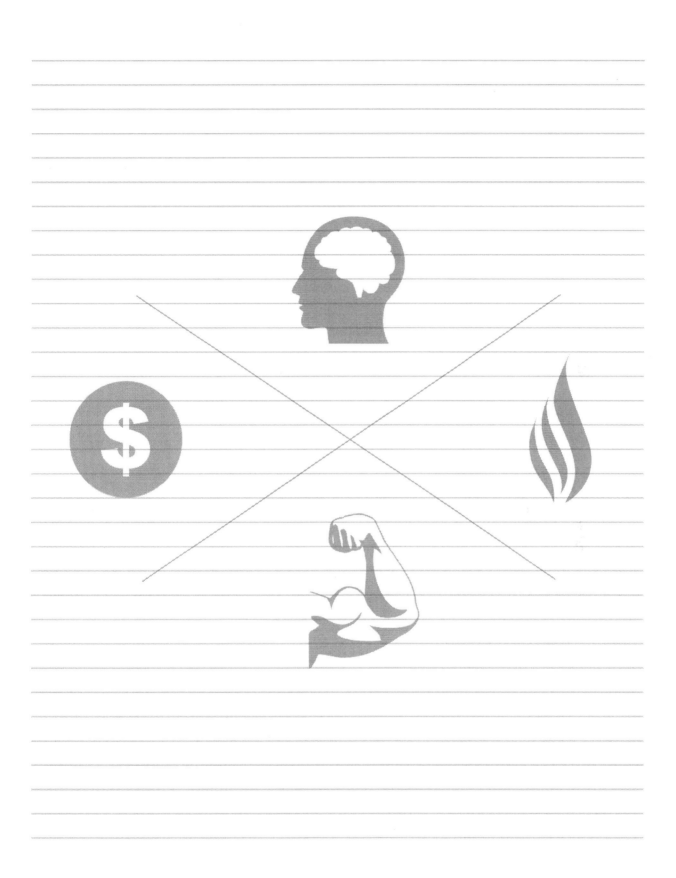

Weekly Wrap-Up

3 great things that happened this week:

_____

_____

_____

4 Futures Score Card

	M	T	W	R	F	S	S	Total	/28
Mind									/7
Meaning									/7
Muscle									/7
Money									/7

Next week, I will improve _____ by...	One area I excelled at this week

Looking Ahead to Next Week...

Major tasks I need to work on

My theme this week is...

Big events coming up that I need to prepare for:	I will improve my 4 Futures Score by doing the following:

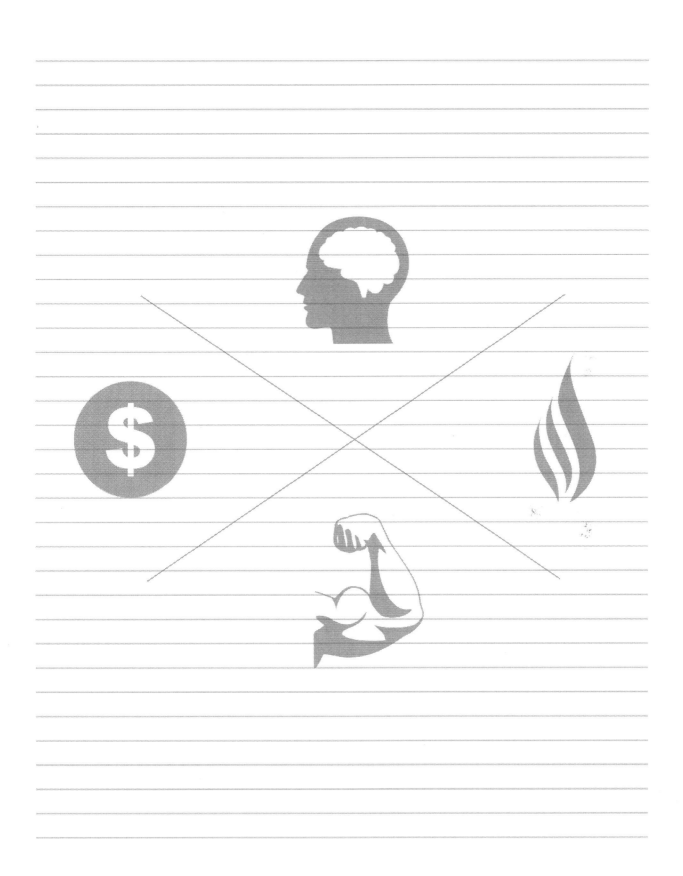

If conscience disapproves, the loudest applauses of the world are of little value. - John Adams

Date _____ / _____ / _____

Daily Priorities:

1 ....
....
....

2 ....
....
....

3 ....
....
....

4 ....
....
....

5 ....
....
....

6 ....
....
....

7 ....
....
....

8 ....
....
....

9 ....
....
....

Today I Appreciate:

1. _____

2. _____

3. _____

I'm strengthened knowing:

I'm looking forward to:

I will enrich my future by...

Mind ☐   ☐ Meaning

Muscle ☐   ☐ Money

When I think of those closest to me...

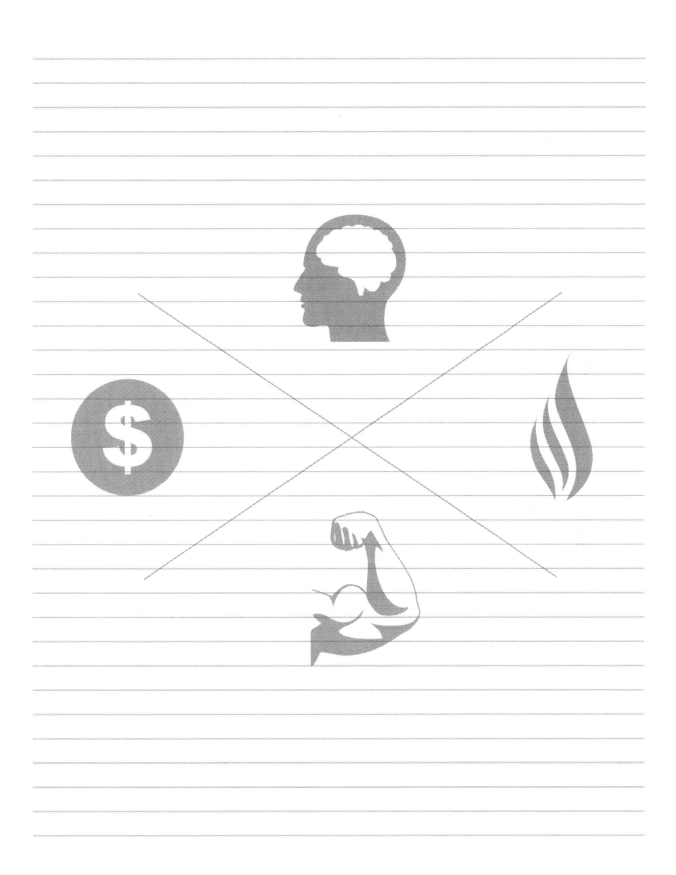

Date _____ / _____ / _____

Daily Priorities:

1 ....
....
....

2 ....
....
....

3 ....
....

4 ....
....
....

5 ....
....
....

6 ....
....

7 ....
....
....

8 ....
....
....

9 ....
....

Today I Appreciate:

1. _____

2. _____

3. _____

I'm strengthened knowing:

I'm looking forward to:

I will enrich my future by...

Mind ☐

☐ Meaning

Muscle ☐

☐ Money

When I think of what money gives me....

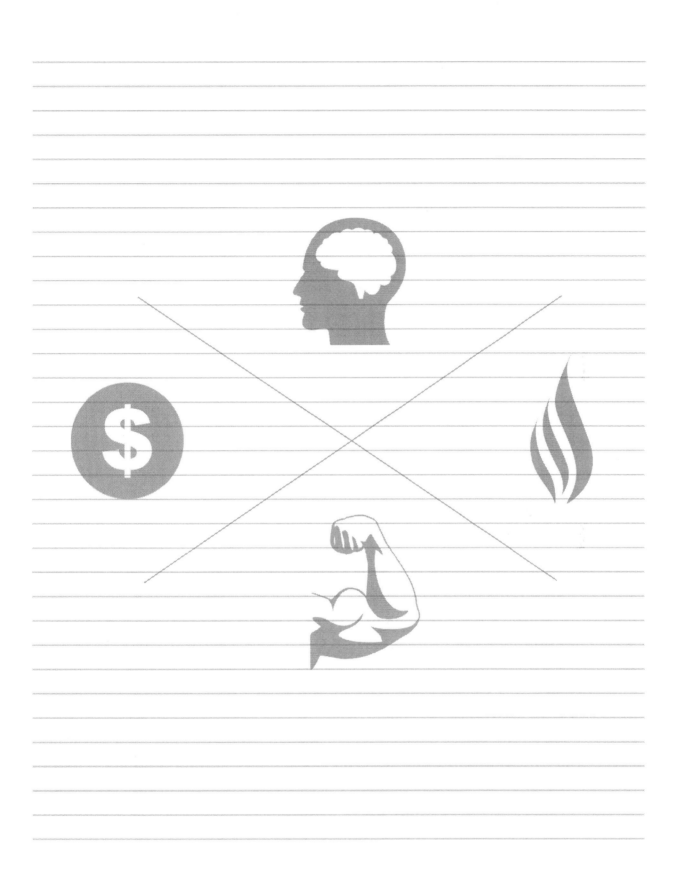

Date _____ / _____ / _____

Daily Priorities:

1 ....

2 ....

3 ....

4 ....

5 ....

6 ....

7 ....

8 ....

9 ....

Today I Appreciate:

1. _____

2. _____

3. _____

I'm strengthened knowing:	I'm looking forward to:

I will enrich my future by...

Mind ☐

☐ Meaning

Muscle ☐

☐ Money

One goal that I am focusing on in my health is…

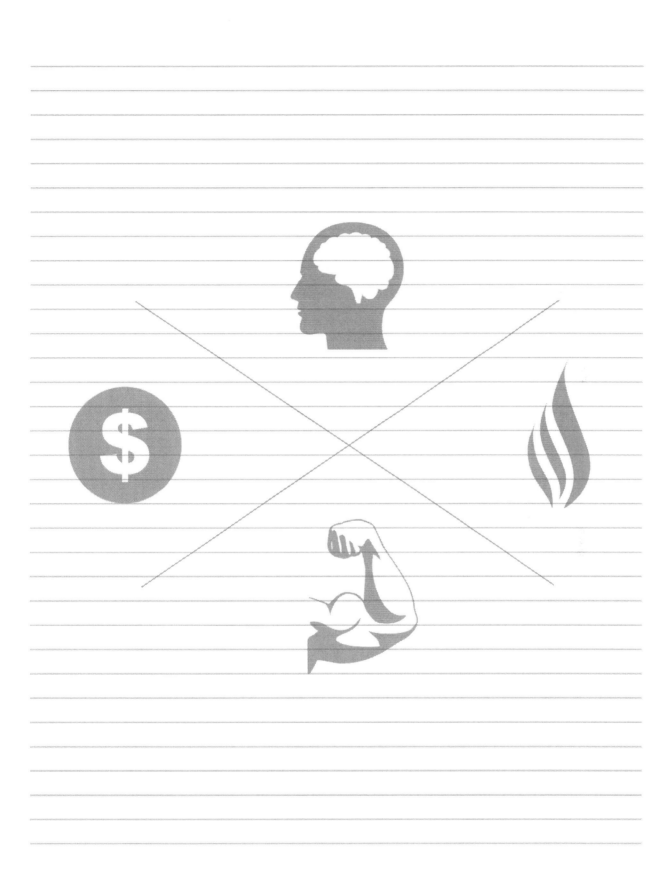

Everything we hear is an opinion, not a fact. Everything we see is a perspective, not the truth. - Marcus Aurelius

Date ___ / ___ / ___

Daily Priorities:

1

2

3

4

5

6

7

8

9

Today I Appreciate:

1. _____

2. _____

3. _____

I'm strengthened knowing:

I'm looking forward to:

I will enrich my future by...

Mind ☐   ☐ Meaning

Muscle ☐   ☐ Money

When stress overtakes my energy, I will try…

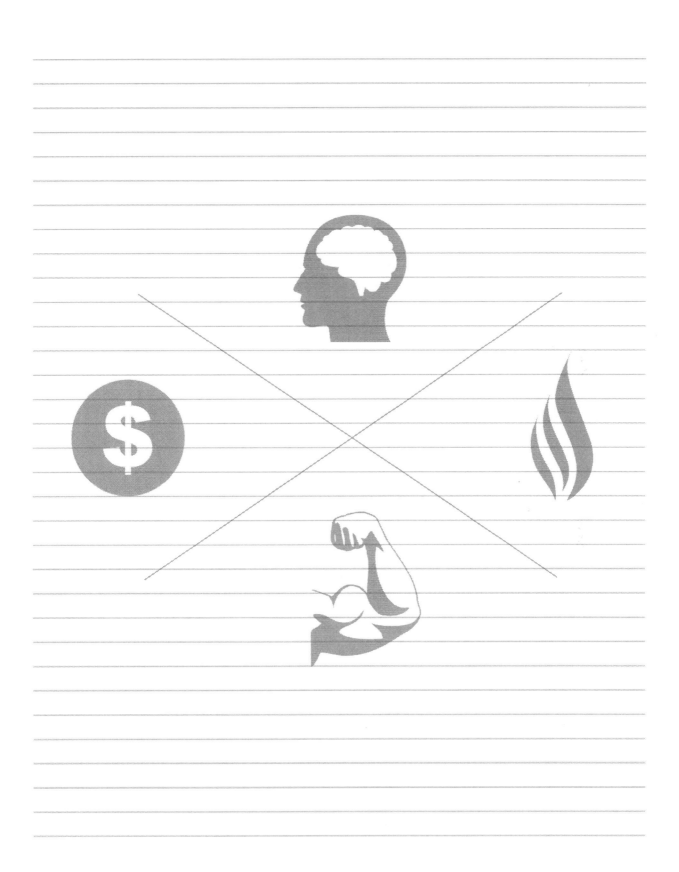

Date ___ / ___ / ___

Daily Priorities:

1

2

3

4

5

6

7

8

9

Today I Appreciate:

1. _____

2. _____

3. _____

I'm strengthened knowing:

I'm looking forward to:

I will enrich my future by...

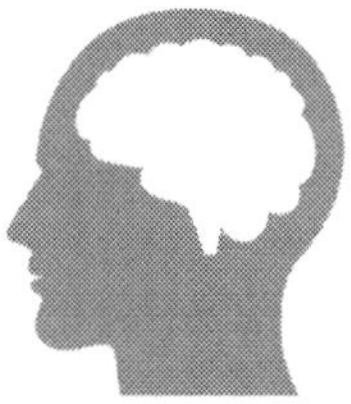

Mind ☐

☐ Meaning

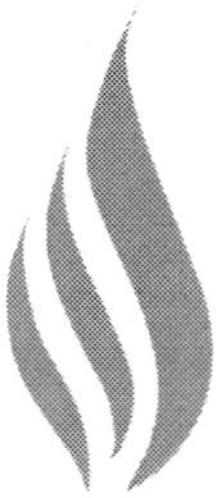

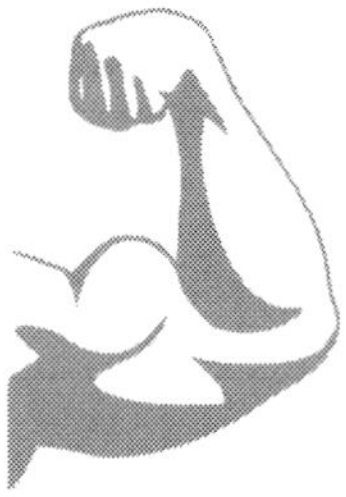

Muscle ☐

☐ Money

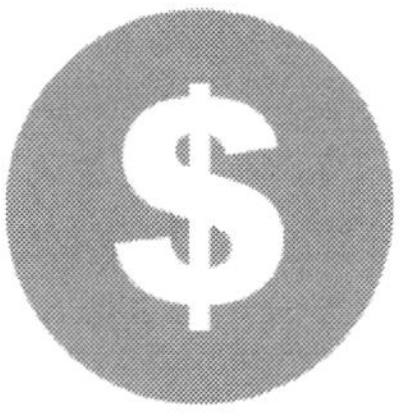

I feel connected to others when...

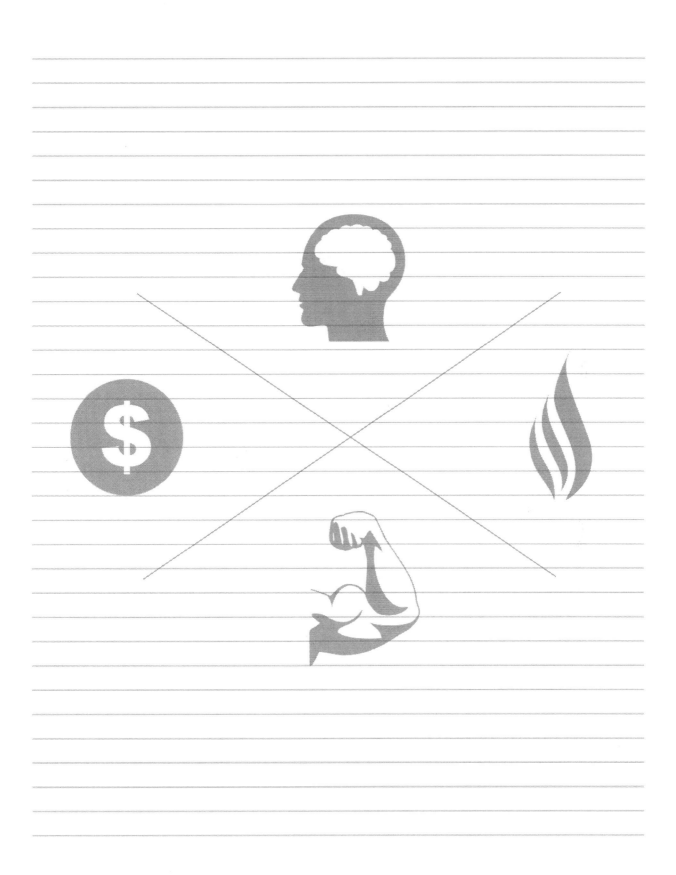

Date _____ / _____ / _____

Today I Appreciate:

1. _____
2. _____
3. _____

Daily Priorities:

1

2

3

4

5

6

7

8

9

I'm strengthened knowing:

I'm looking forward to:

I will enrich my future by...

Mind ☐

☐ Meaning

Muscle ☐

☐ Money

I will avoid focusing too much on money by...

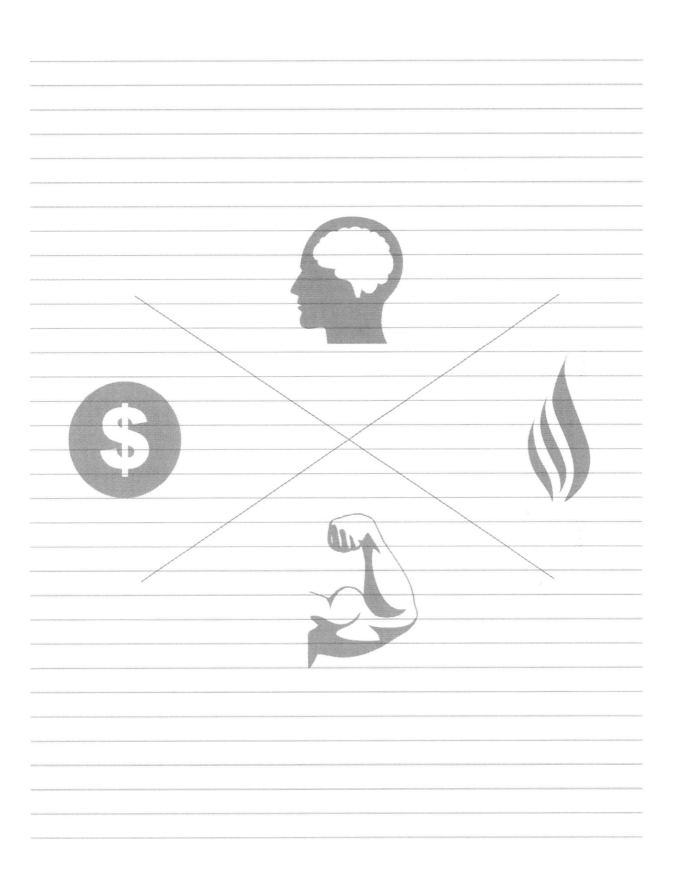

Date ____ / ____ / ____

Today I Appreciate:

1. _____

2. _____

3. _____

Daily Priorities:

1 ....

2 ....

3 ....

4 ....

5 ....

6 ....

7 ....

8 ....

9 ....

I'm strengthened knowing:

I'm looking forward to:

I will enrich my future by...

Mind ☐

☐ Meaning

Muscle ☐

☐ Money

I often feel physically my best when…

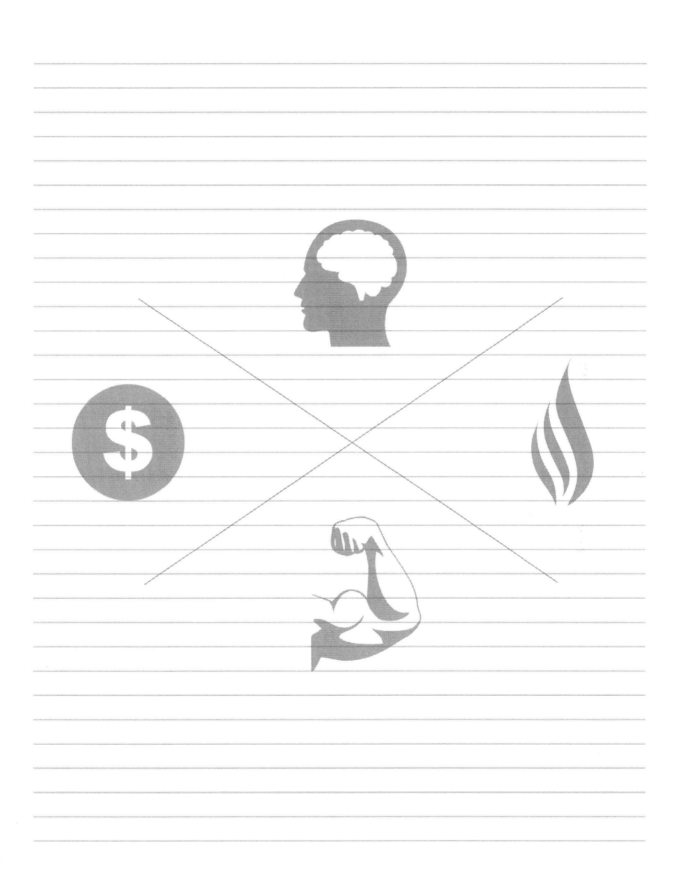

Weekly Wrap-Up

3 great things that happened this week:

_____

_____

_____

4 Futures Score Card

	M	T	W	R	F	S	S	Total	/28
Mind									/7
Meaning									/7
Muscle									/7
Money									/7

Next week, I will improve _____ by...	One area I excelled at this week

Looking Ahead to Next Week...

Major tasks I need to work on

My theme this week is...

Big events coming up that I need to prepare for:	I will improve my 4 Futures Score by doing the following:

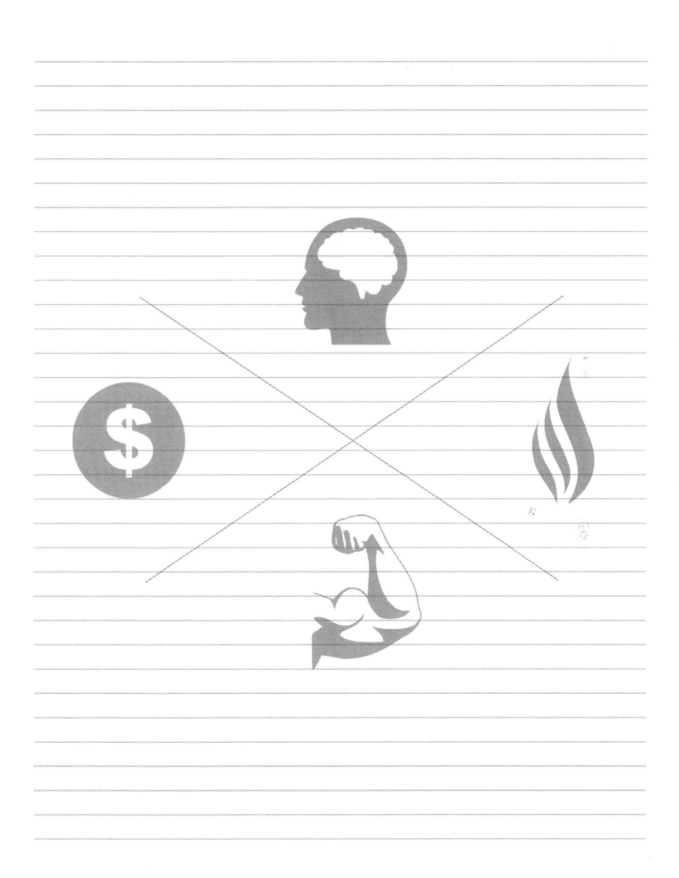

Time Journal

This addition to the 4 Futures Journal is meant to help you realize how time can be better used in your day. In our private-client meetings, we usually recommend doing this once per quarter or more. We give you 4 days here to follow the practice.

Instructions:
- Write down what you do in each 30-minute segment. If you do multiple activities, write them all clearly and separately.
- Complete the exercise for 4 days in a row.
- At the end, go back and mark times with:

• Critical: Put [Square markings] around activities that are critical, and only you can do.

• Critical for Someone Else: Underline any activities that while important, can possibly be delegated to someone else to complete

• Low Impact: Put a **mid-line crossout** through any activities that are unproductive and that have no value in your life and goals

- After marking up your time journal, review to see how much time is spent doing Critical versus Low Impact activities. Think about how much more productive you could be if you cut out the worthless activities.

- Review how many activities you currently do, but could possibly delegate. Consider what hiring a part-time personal assistant could do for your life if you could out-source these low-value activities.

Example Time Journal

TIME JOURNAL

Todays Date: 8/17/19

Time	Tasks
4:30AM	4:45 [wake up, coffee, meditate, journal]
5:30AM	[Run, Shower] ~~Checked Facebook and email~~
6:30AM	wake up kids, get ready for school, drive to school
7:30AM	Drive to work [AM huddle, Start Clinical work]
8:30AM	[Office work & patient Care]
9:30AM	[Patient Care]
10:30AM	[Patient Care]
11:30AM	lunch, checked emails, worked on documents [3-min meditation]
12:30PM	[Patient Care]
1:30PM	[Patient Care]
2:30PM	[Patient Care]
3:30PM	[Patient Care]
4:30PM	[Wrapped up notes, planned for tomorrow]
5:30PM	drive home, dinner - prep. and eat w/ family [2-min. mindfulness]
6:30PM	Play w/ kids, Go get icecream
7:30PM	Put kids to bed, bath, ~~read news on phone~~
8:30PM	Clean up kitchen, sweep floors, answer emails
9:30PM	[Prepare for bed] [EOD Journal] watch TV show with wife.
10:30PM	Sleep
11:30PM	Sleep
12:30AM	Sleep

TIME JOURNAL

Todays Date: _____

Time	Tasks
4:30AM	
5:30AM	
6:30AM	
7:30AM	
8:30AM	
9:30AM	
10:30AM	
11:30AM	
12:30PM	
1:30PM	
2:30PM	
3:30PM	
4:30PM	
5:30PM	
6:30PM	
7:30PM	
8:30PM	
9:30PM	
10:30PM	
11:30PM	
12:30AM	

TIME JOURNAL

Todays Date: _____

Time	Tasks
4:30AM	
5:30AM	
6:30AM	
7:30AM	
8:30AM	
9:30AM	
10:30AM	
11:30AM	
12:30PM	
1:30PM	
2:30PM	
3:30PM	
4:30PM	
5:30PM	
6:30PM	
7:30PM	
8:30PM	
9:30PM	
10:30PM	
11:30PM	
12:30AM	

TIME JOURNAL

Todays Date: _____

Time	Tasks
4:30AM	
5:30AM	
6:30AM	
7:30AM	
8:30AM	
9:30AM	
10:30AM	
11:30AM	
12:30PM	
1:30PM	
2:30PM	
3:30PM	
4:30PM	
5:30PM	
6:30PM	
7:30PM	
8:30PM	
9:30PM	
10:30PM	
11:30PM	
12:30AM	

TIME JOURNAL

Todays Date: _____

Time	Tasks
4:30AM	
5:30AM	
6:30AM	
7:30AM	
8:30AM	
9:30AM	
10:30AM	
11:30AM	
12:30PM	
1:30PM	
2:30PM	
3:30PM	
4:30PM	
5:30PM	
6:30PM	
7:30PM	
8:30PM	
9:30PM	
10:30PM	
11:30PM	
12:30AM	

Made in the USA
Monee, IL
07 October 2021

46f5e79d-a2bb-4304-9720-cdd31ee9fab0R01